"While only one day of the year is dedicated solely to honoring our veterans, Americans must never forget the sacrifices that many of our fellow countrymen have made to defend our country and protect our freedoms." – Randy Neugebauer

The number of veterans residing in Arizona is quite staggering. But with all of the benefits and entitlements that Arizona has to offer its veterans, it's no wonder why they decide to make Arizona their home.

Arizona has a total of 532,206 veterans statewide.

Male - 477,985
Female - 54,221

War-time Veterans - 425,067

Gulf War - 159,896
Vietnam Era - 185,867
Korean Conflict - 53,727
World War II - 25,577

Peace-time Veterans - 107,139

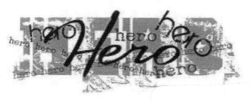

"OUR DEBT TO THE

HEROIC MEN AND VALIANT

WOMEN IN THE SERVICE

OF OUR COUNTRY CAN

NEVER BE REPAID. THEY

HAVE EARNED OUR

UNDYING GRATITUDE.

AMERICA WILL NEVER FORGET

THEIR SACRIFICES."

- President Harry S. Truman

Veterans State Benefits Arizona

The Ultimate Guide to

Your Hard-Earned Veterans Benefits

By: Derek Simmons

Active Military, Retirees, and
Disabled Retired Veterans
State and Local Benefits and
Entitlements

These are _YOUR_ Benefits and Entitlements.

You've _EARNED_ them! So, go and some fun!

Enjoy!!

Limit of Liability and Disclaimer of Warranty

The Author is only aware of the material presented within this book. The Author has compiled this information to the best of his ability and makes the point that what is presented herein, is by no way all and everything that is available in the way of benefits for the active duty military, the retired veteran or the retired veteran with disabilities. The Author has done his due diligence in verifying the information herein. The Author does not endorse any business, organization or website mentioned in this book. Readers should be aware that internet websites listed in this book may have changed or disappeared between when this book was written and when it is read. Most of the information in this publication was obtained from the World Wide Web, freely and without malicious intent. The Author has no desire to harm nor hurt any of the businesses or organizations listed within this publication. The information you see was retrieved either by the Author visiting the website listed for each business or organization, or by calling the businesses or organizations at the phone number that is provided for them, or by the Author visiting most of the businesses himself.

Information was received and applied to this publication by the Author. The Author admits to finding and using the websites listed in this publication and has used some of the information listed on said websites. The information provided herein is for your personal, non-commercial use. You may not sell or otherwise exchange the contents, in part or in whole, for anything of value. You may not use the information of this publication for advertising nor in any commercial venture. All businesses and organizations and services mentioned in this publication are for informational purposes only. No endorsements are made or implied, nor is the absence of company or trade name in this publication to be construed as a discouragement. The Author of this publication has not patronized all of the businesses or organizations or websites and services listed so, ***caveat emptor.***

BOOK DEDICATION

This book was written for all the men and women currently serving in the United States Armed Forces and for all my fellow veterans. I humbly offer my most sincere gratitude, appreciation, and respect to you all. Without your sacrifice, dedication, and loyalty to our country, this book, nor freedom of expression, would not be possible.

For over two centuries, Americans have fought and died to protect and defend the integrity and ideals of the Constitution of the United States of America. Since the American Revolution, over 45 million veterans have served; more than one million have died in the name of Freedom. Many others have made enormous sacrifices, suffered greatly, and experienced unknowable loss, so that we all could live a better life.

It is my mission to provide you with the most comprehensive, up to date, informative, one of a kind information available on veterans' benefits. I strive to support every veteran with clear and responsible data. This never before published information is designed to help you obtain the maximum in veterans' benefits from the state of Arizona and its local agencies and businesses. I am devoted to helping Arizona residents that are currently serving and all that have served, to the fullest.

This is not your typical "Here's Your Veterans Benefits" kind of book. The Author wanted something different. There are a lot of "Benefits Books" flooding the market right now. The Author has tried a new approach to find your benefits, by contacting local agencies and businesses throughout the State of Arizona and has brought to light some of the best benefits and entitlements that Arizona has to offer their veterans. Now, not all the benefits and entitlements listed in this book are in Arizona, but they needed to be mentioned.

This book is dedicated to the many heroic men and valiant women who've paid the ultimate price for freedom while serving faithfully, with courage, honor, dedication and much sacrifice. So, go enjoy yourself, have some fun, you've earned it!

Contents at a Glance

Introduction

If you are reading this book, there is a real good chance that you are a military veteran, or you have a family member or friend that is a veteran.

There are numerous benefits for those that have served or are currently serving our great country. Most veterans are aware of what Federal benefits there are, and how to receive them. This book does not cover "those benefits"- instead, this book covers those benefits that the state of Arizona proudly offers its veterans, to show their gratitude and appreciation for your dedication and sacrifice.

You do not have to read this book cover to cover to understand these benefits. You might only be interested in one or two types of benefits or maybe a select few. Feel free to read at your leisure through the sections that most interest you. My guess, every section will get you excited enough to read the entire book!

No matter where you start, I wish you all the best in finding the benefit(s) that you want to explore – ***you have definitely earned them!!***

From a fellow veteran, I want to say thank you for your service, your dedication, your courage, and your sacrifice to our country.

"Honor to the Soldier and Sailor
everywhere, who bravely bears his
country's cause. Honor, also, to the
citizen who cares for his brother in
the field and serves, as he best can,
the same cause."

– Abraham Lincoln

Wounded Warrior Benefits

State Tax Advantage: Military retirement payments and/or survivor benefits up to $2,500.00 per year are exempt. Compensation received for active service as a member of the Armed Forces of the United States for any month during any part of which members served in a combat zone is exempt. eligibility: Retiree for retired pay exemption and any Armed Forces Service Member serving in a combat zone for combat pay exemption.

Property Tax

Persons who are on active duty in military service and are absent from the state, or those confined in any licensed hospital, may submit an eligibility affidavit certified by any authorized official. Any person applying for exemption from taxation by reason of military service shall, before application is made, record their discharge papers with the county recorder in the county where the application is made. The exemption applies first to real estate, then to a mobile home or automobile.

"The United States flag does not fly
because the wind moves past it....
The United States flag flies from the
last breath of each military member
who has died protecting it."

Exemption of property tax for widows and widowers

Exemption for property of widows, widowers and disabled persons are outlined in A.R.S.§ 42-11111 as follows:

A). The property of widows, widowers and disabled persons who are residents of this state is exempt from taxation to the extent allowed by Article IX, Sections 2, 2.1, 2.2 and 2.3, Constitution of Arizona, and subject to the conditions and limitations prescribed by this section.

B). Pursuant to Article IX, Section 2.3, Constitution of Arizona, the exemptions from taxation under this section are allowed in the amount of:

1. Three thousand dollars if the person's total assessment does not exceed twenty thousand dollars.

2. No exemption if the person's total assessment exceeds twenty thousand dollars

C). On or before December 31 of each year, the department shall increase the following amounts based on the average annual percentage increase, if any, in the GDP price deflator in the two most recent complete state fiscal years:

The total allowable exemption amount and the total assessment limitation amount under subsection B of this section.

The total income limitation amounts under subsection E, paragraphs 1 and 2 of this section. For the purposes of this subsection, "GDP price deflator" means the average of the four implicit price deflators for the gross domestic product reported by the United States Department of Commerce or its successor for the four quarters of the state fiscal year.

D). For the purpose of determining the amount of the allowable exemption pursuant to subsection B of the section, the person's total assessment shall not include the value of any vehicle that is taxed under Title 28, Chapter 16, Article 3.

NOTE: The exemption is applied to real estate first, then to mobile home or an automobile. Please call your County Assessor's Office for more assistance.

Disabled Persons

An exemption from property taxation is available to any persons who, after age 17 has been medically certified as totally and permanently disabled in the year immediately preceding the year for which the applicant applies. The income from all sources of a disabled person and their spouse, together with the income from all sources of any children residing with the disabled person shall not exceed $13,200 if there are no children under the age of 18 with the applicant, or $18,840 if one or more of the applicant's children under the age of 18 is certified as being totally and permanently disabled, either physically or mentally. Contact your County Assessor's office for eligibility.

Military Disability Retired Pay

Retirees who entered the military before September 24, 1975, and members receiving disability retirements based on combat injuries or who could receive disability payments from the Veterans Administration are covered by laws giving disability broad exemption from federal income tax. Most military retired pay based on service-related disabilities also is free from federal income tax, but there is no guarantee of total protection. Contact your local IRS Regional office for the latest laws concerning this exemption.

Military SPP/SSPP/RC SPP RS FPP: Is generally

subject to state taxes for those states with income tax. Check with state Department of Revenue.

Vehicle License Tax and Registration Fees

A Veteran residing in Arizona shall be exempt from a vehicle license tax (VLT) on a vehicle acquired by the veteran through financial aid from the U.S. Department of Veterans Affairs. A.R.S. § 28-5802(A)(1).

No VLT or registration fee shall be collected from any veteran for a personally owned vehicle is such veteran is certified by the U.S. Department of Veterans Affairs to be 100% service-connected disabled and drawing compensation on that basis. A.R.S. § 28-5802(A)(2).

Until the surviving spouse of a 100% disabled veteran remarries or dies, the law also applies to the survivor. The U.S. Department of Veterans Affairs will provide the attached certification letter to all eligible spouses upon request. To receive the VLT and registration fee exemptions, the eligible spouse must present this certification letter to the Division at the time of vehicle registration. A new certification will be required each year.

A veteran claiming an exemption prescribed shall present satisfactory proof of such U.S. Department of Veterans Affairs financial aid or government compensation and certificate of determination of one hundred percent disability, as applicable.

Such exemption may be claimed and granted during each 12-month period for only one vehicle or any replacement of such vehicle owned by the veteran. A.R.S. §28-5802(B).

No license tax or registration fee shall be collected from any veteran for a personally owned or co-owned vehicle if such veteran is certified by the U.S. Department of Veterans Affairs to be 100 % service-connected disabled and drawing compensation on that basis. A veteran residing in Arizona claiming an exemption shall provide satisfactory proof of U.S. Department of Veterans Affairs disability compensation of a 100% disability. Such exemption may be claimed and granted during each 12-month period for only one vehicle or any replacement of such vehicle that is owned by the veteran. The exemption also applies to the surviving spouse, until remarriage, and to only one vehicle or any replacement of the vehicle owned by the veteran or the surviving spouse.

Veteran designation is now available for Arizona Drivers Licenses and Identification Cards.

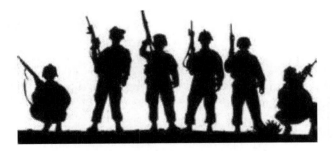

Special Vehicle License Plates

Congressional Medal of Honor Plate - A Medal of Honor plate is issued free of charge and there are no other applicable costs to the veteran.

Former Prisoner of War Plate - A Former P.O.W. plate is issued to persons qualifying as former prisoners of war. Does not grant special parking privileges. A $15.00 additional fee in addition to all applicable licensing fees is charged, and a $5.00 for annual renewal. The initial application fee goes to the State Home for Veterans trust fund. Eligibility: Applicant must have been captured and incarcerated by an enemy of the U.S. during a period of conflict with the U.S., have received an honorable discharge and provide a copy of a current membership from the American Ex- Prisoners of War Association, or an original letter from the Arizona Department of Veterans Services (ADVS) verifying eligibility. May also be issued to the spouse, parent, child, brother, or sister of an eligible person who has been issued the plate.

Purple Heart Plate - A Purple Heart plate is issued to persons qualifying as Purple Heart recipient for a $25.00 additional fee in addition to all other applicable licensing fees, and $5.00 for annual renewal. The initial application fee goes to the State Home for Veterans trust fund. Eligibility: Applicant must be a veteran and a Purple Heart Medal recipient, and provide a copy of a DD214 or 215, WDAGO forms 53 – 55, NAVPERS 553 or NAVMC 78, which indicates PURPLE Heart Medal recipient or provide an original letter from the Arizona Department of Veterans Services verifying eligibility. May also be issued to the spouse, parent, child, brother, or sister of an eligible person who has been issued the plate.

Pearl Harbor Survivors Plate - Any resident
of Arizona who was a member of the Armed Forces of the United States, received an honorable discharge, and was stationed at Pearl Harbor, the island of Oahu (or offshore not exceeding 3 miles), on December 7, 1941, during the hours of 7:55 A.M. and 9:45 A.M., is eligible for a Pearl Harbor Survivor plate. An initial fee of $25.00 is charged in addition to the registration fee with an annual renewal fee of $5.00. The initial application fee goes to the State Home for Veterans trust fund.

Eligibility: Veteran must have received an honorable discharge and needs to provide Form 02-25, Part II from the Arizona Department of Veterans Services. May also be issued to the spouse, parent, child, brother, or sister of an eligible person who has been issued this plate.

Gold Star Family Plate - A Gold Star plate may be

obtained at an initial cost of $25.00 with a $25.00 annual renewal fee. $17.00 of the fee goes toward the construction and maintenance of the Enduring Freedom Memorial. Eligibility: Applicant must be a spouse or (by adoption or blood) a child, parent, brother, or sister of a person who lost his or her life while on active duty in the U.S, Armed Forces.

National Guard Plate - Any resident of Arizona who

is or has been a member of the Arizona National Guard or Arizona Air National Guard may apply for a distinctive number plate. An initial and renewal fee of $25.00 is charged in addition to the registration fee. $17.00 of the initial and annual fee goes to the Arizona National Guard morale, welfare, and recreation fund. Eligibility: National Guard service member and certificate of eligibility required when submitting DMV application. May also be issued to the spouse of an eligible person.

Veteran Plate - Any resident of Arizona who was a member

of U.S. Armed Forces and received an honorable discharge may apply for a distinctive number plate. An initial and renewal fee of $25.00 is charged in addition to the registration fee. $17.00 of the initial and renewal fee goes to a special fund to benefit veterans in Arizona. Eligibility: Must be a veteran and provide a copy of a DD214 215, 2A, 2(retired), 2(reserve), or 1173; or provide an original statement of honorable service from the U.S. Department of Veterans Affairs or the Arizona Department of Veterans Services or any one of the following cards: American Legion, Disabled American Veterans, Military Officers of America, Veterans Administration Medical, Veterans of Foreign Wars, Military of Purple Heart, Vietnam Veterans of America, Active duty or Inactive duty.

May also be issued to the spouse, parent, child, brother, or sister of an eligible person who has been issued the plate.

Military Spouse/Freedom Plate - Anyone
may purchase the Freedom plate for a cost of $25.00 in addition to all other applicable licensing fees. A renewable fee of $25.00 is incurred. $17.00 goes to a special fund to benefit veterans in Arizona.

Automatic Military Extension / 5-year license - If the expiration date on a driver's
license of an active duty military member expires while on active duty, the license will remain valid for up to 6 months from the time the member leaves military service. Military personnel and dependents stationed in Arizona may also apply for a 5-year license.

Disabled Veteran License Tax Exemption - A veteran owning or co-owning a vehicle is
exempt from payment of VLT or registration fee, if the veteran is certified by the U.S. Department of Veterans Affairs to be 100% disabled and drawing compensation on that basis. The exemption also applies to the surviving spouse, until remarriage, and to only one vehicle or any replacement of the vehicle owned by the veteran or the surviving spouse.

Tax and Registration Fees Exemption
The Direction of the Department of Transportation shall provide a one-year exemption for vehicle licensing tax (VLT) and registration fees and implement measures to expedite services to military personnel while engaged in active duty. Motor vehicles owned or leased must be currently registered in Arizona in the member's name on the date he or she received orders to active military duty. This exemption allows the registration of a motor vehicle to be renewed for one year without payment of the VLT and registration fees.

Military Discharge Documentation –
Shall be recorded by any County Recorder, free of charge. Contact your County Recorder's Office for more information.

Employment Preferences - Age Limit: An Honorably discharged veteran shall be eligible for employment preference, rights, and privileges under any merit system in the state or any political subdivision thereof, regardless of age, if otherwise qualified.

Civil Service: Veterans who pass an examination for employment by the state, county, or city will have 5 points added to their certification score. The veteran must have served for more than six (6) months and be separated under honorable conditions. Veterans entitled to compensation for a service-connected disability will have 19 points added to their certification score. Certain spouses or surviving spouses shall be given a 5-point preference if the veteran died of a service-connected disability.

Fire Department: Members of any fire company inducted into the military establishment of the United States for military training are authorized reinstatement to their previous rating after discharge from military service.

Police and Fire Department: The period of military service shall be included in computing the length of service of the employee to determine eligibility for retirement.

Reserve Status/War Emergency: Appointive officers or employees of the state or of a political subdivision will be reinstated to their former position upon completion of military service to which he or she was inducted or ordered during time of war or was called to active service because of their status as an active or inactive member of the Reserves.

Professional and Occupational Licenses:
Every funeral director, embalmer, or apprentice embalmer who serves in the Armed Forces during a time of war is exempt from paying renewal license fees for the duration of the war and six months thereafter or for a period of six months following discharge from the Armed Forces.

Additional Benefits Available for Service-Connected Disabled Veterans

0% TO 20%

- ➢ Certificate of Eligibility for home loan guarantee
- ➢ Home loan guarantee user fee exemption
- ➢ VA priority medical treatment card
- ➢ Vocational Rehabilitation and Counseling under Title 38 USC, Chapter 31, (must be at least 10%)
- ➢ Service-Disabled Veterans Insurance (Maximum of $10,000 coverage), must be filed within 2 years from date of NEW service connection
- ➢ Ten-point Civil Service preference (10 points added to Civil Service test score)
- ➢ Clothing Allowance for veterans who use or wear a prosthetic or orthopedic appliance (artificial limb, brace, wheelchair) or used prescribed medications for skin condition which tends to wear, tear, or soil clothing
- ➢ Temporary total evaluation (100%) based upon hospitalization for a service-connected disability in excess of 21 days; or surgical treatment for a service-connected disability necessitating at least one month of convalescence or immobilization by cast, without surgery of one or more major joints

30% IN ADDITION TO THE ABOVE:

- ▪ Additional allowance for dependent spouse, child(ren), step-child(ren), helpless child(ren), full-time students, between the ages of 18 and 23 and parent(s)
- ▪ Additional allowance for a spouse who is a patient in a nursing home or helpless or blind or so nearly helpless or blind as to require the regular aid and attendance of another person
- ▪ Non-competitive Federal employment

40% *IN ADDITION TO THE ABOVE:*

- o Automobile grant and/or special adaptive equipment for an automobile provided there is loss or permanent loss of use of one or both feet; loss or permanent loss of one or both hands or permanent impaired vision of both eyes with central visual acuity or 20/200 or less in better eye
- o Special Adaptive equipment may also be applied for if there is ankylosis of one or both knees or one or both hips
- o VA medical outpatient treatment for any condition except dental
- o Preventive health care services
- o Hospital care and medical services in non-VA facilities under an authorized fee basis agreement

60% IN ADDITION TO THE ABOVE:

- • Increased compensation (100%) based on individual unemployability (applies to veterans who are unable to obtain or maintain substantially gainful employment due to service-connected disability)

100% IN ADDITION TO THE ABOVE:

- ❖ Dental treatment: Waiver of National Service Life Insurance total disability income provisions
- ❖ Veterans employment preference for spouse
- ❖ Specially Adaptive Housing for veterans who have loss or permanent loss of use of both lower extremities or blindness in both eyes having light only plus loss or permanent loss of one lower extremity or the loss or permanent loss of one lower extremity with loss or permanent loss of use of one upper extremity or loss or permanent loss of use of one extremity together with an organic disease which affects the function of balance and propulsion as to preclude locomotion without the aid of braces, crutches, canes, or wheelchair

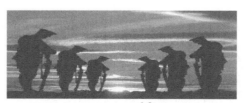

10

- ❖ Special Home Adaptation Grant (for veterans who don't qualify for Specially Adapted Housing) may be applied for if the veteran is permanently and totally disabled to blindness in both eyes with visual acuity of 5/200 or less of the loss or permanent loss of use of both hands
- ❖ Department of Defense Commissary privileges

100% PERMANENT AND TOTAL - IN ADDITION TO THE ABOVE:

- ❖ Civilian Health and Medical Program for dependents and survivors (CHAMPVA)
- ❖ Survivors and dependents education assistance under Title 38 USC Chapter 35

HUNTING AND FISHING PRIVILEGES

Resident hunting and fishing licenses for members of the Armed Forces on active duty, stationed in state are available upon application. Complimentary licenses may be granted to veterans 70 years or older who have been residing in Arizona for at least 25 years. Complimentary licenses will be issued to veterans that are verified by the U.S. Department of Veterans Affairs to be 100% service–connected disabled and who have been a resident for one year or more. Contact the nearest Department of Game and Fish office for more information.

A.R.S. 15-1802: IN-STATE TUITION FOR HONORABLY DISCHARGED VETERANS

Beginning in the fall semester of 2011, a person who is honorably discharged from the Armed Forces of the United States shall be granted immediate classification as an in-state student on honorable discharge from the armed forces and, while in continuous attendance toward the degree for which currently enrolled, does not lose in-state student classification if the person has met the following requirements:

1. Registered to vote in this state

2. Demonstrated objective evidence of intent to be a resident of Arizona that, for the purposes of this section, includes at least one of the following:

   (a) An Arizona driver license.
   (b) Arizona motor vehicle registration.
   (c) Employment history in Arizona.
   (d) Transfer of major banking services to Arizona.
   (e) Change of permanent address on all pertinent record
   (f). Other materials of whatever kind or source relevant to domicile or residency status.

Troops to Teachers: State Offices provide participants with counseling and assistance regarding certification requirements, routes to state certification and employment leads. Pending availability of funds, financial assistance may be provided to eligible individuals.

Arizona Educational Benefits

National Guard Tuition Assistance: The

maximum amount available per Arizona National guard member for State Education Priority Reimbursement for tuition is $250.00 per semester hour, not to exceed an annual cap of $6,500.00 per state fiscal year (July 1 – June 30). Eligibility: National Guard service member

Tuition and Fees–Deferred Payment: A Veteran or

eligible dependent who has applied for educational benefits under the G.I. Bill state-supported community colleges, colleges, or universities may defer payment of tuition, fees and required books f or a period of 120 days with no interest charges. If, at the end of such period, the person has not yet received from the U.S. Department of Veterans Affairs, the initial benefit monies for tuition and fees, an extension may be granted until such time benefits are received.

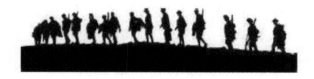

Other Benefits

Burial and Headstones: When a Veteran or a surviving spouse dies without sufficient means for funeral expenses, the County Board of Supervisors is responsible to ensure that burial will not be in a portion of the ground used exclusively for burial of paupers. A suitable plot will be used, and the county may apply to the U.S. Department of Veterans Affairs for expenses not to exceed $150.00.

When the county buries an indigent veteran, the county clerk will make an application to the U.S. Department of Veterans Affairs for a suitable headstone and make arrangements for it to be placed at the head of the grave.

Memorial Bronze Markers: For individuals or groups, are furnished for eligible deceased active duty service members and Veterans whose remains are not recovered or identified, are buried at sea, donated to science or whose cremated remains have been scattered. Eligibility: Any Veteran who has other than a dishonorable discharge s eligible for burial. Spouses and certain dependents are also eligible for burial. There is no charge for interment for veterans and a onetime nominal fee of $300.00 for eligible spouses and dependents.

Voting in Elections: Absentee registration and voting by active duty military personnel and their eligible dependents residing outside of the state may be accomplished by prior to 7:00 pm on an election day. The County Recorder may accept a federal postcard application in lieu of an affidavit of registration.

Recording of Discharges: Any County Recorder, free of charge shall record military discharge papers. Location of each County Recorder's Office may be found in the blue pages of your local area phone directory.

Public Record Certification: Public officials shall issue without charge, certified copies of public records for use in making a claim for pension, compensation, allotment allowance, insurance, or other benefits from the United States.

Credit for Military Service for State Retirement Benefits:

A participant of the state system or plan may receive credited past service or future service for active military service if the participant was honorably discharged from service.

The period of military service for which the participant receives credited service is not on account with any other retirement system. Contact the nearest state personnel office for additional information and eligibility.

Arizona Department of Veterans' Services

"Valor is stability, not of legs and arms, but of courage and the soul." – Michel de Montaigne

Enriching and Honoring Arizona's Veterans and their Families through Education, Advocacy, and Service

The Arizona Department of Veterans' Services (ADVS) Arizona has provided services to Arizona Veterans since 1925, when it created the position of Veterans' Service Officer. This position was abolished in 1951 and replaced by the Arizona Veterans' Service Commission. In 1973, the Commission was integrated into the Department of Economic Security. Primarily at the request of various Veterans' organizations, the Governor reestablished the Commission as a separate agency in 1982. In 1999, the Legislature separated the Commission from the agency by making the Commission an advisory body and creating a separate Arizona Department of Veterans' Services headed by a governor-appointed director.

The ADVS provides direct services to Veterans through the administration of 15 Veterans Benefits Offices throughout the state - helping Veterans connect with their VA benefits, two skilled-nursing Veterans' Home facilities in Phoenix and Tucson that provide short and long-term care, one Veterans' Memorial Cemetery in Sierra Vista with additional cemeteries under development in Northern Arizona at Camp Navajo and Southern Arizona in Marana - north of Tucson, along with Fiduciary services to provide conservator and guardian services for incapacitated Veterans.

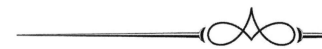

In addition, the ADVS provides critical, state-wide coordination and technical assistance to services and organizations serving Veterans. This includes activities such as coordinating services across private and public sectors in serving targeted populations such as Veterans experiencing homelessness, and special needs for the growing population of Women Veterans - many of whom are at-risk, as well as building community capacity to address Veteran employment and higher education.

There are AVDS offices all throughout the state. Just visit their website to find an office that is closest to where you are, and they are always glad to assist you in whatever it is that you might need - www.dvs.az.gov

VETERANS' EMPLOYMENT RESOURCES

The Arizona Department of Veterans' Services has partnered with the Arizona Coalition for Military Families to connect service members, veterans and their family members to employment, educational and small business ownership opportunities. The Military/Veteran Employment Portal includes:

Military Skills Translator – Translates your service's MOS, AFSC or Rating skill set and responsibilities into civilian HR terms

Online Resume Builder – Builds a competitive civilian resume based on the skills you acquired in the military

Online Document Storage – Store and retrieve your resumes and cover letters online

Personalized Job Portal – Jobs matching your experience and qualifications are sent to you automatically. The Military/Veteran Employment Portal is part of the Military/Veteran Employment Resource Center located at the Arizona National Guard Personnel Readiness Center at Papago Park Military Reservation (52nd Street and McDowell in Phoenix).

Military/Veteran Employment Resource Center
1335 N. 52nd Street
Phoenix, AZ 85008
602-267-2534

The Military/Veteran Employment Resource Center is open to all service members, veterans & their families.

VETERAN'S PROGRAM

DES operates two programs throughout Arizona to assist veterans in finding employment:

Disabled Veterans Outreach Program (DVOP): DVOP specialists provide intensive services to meet the employment needs of special disabled veterans, disabled veterans, veterans and eligible persons.

DVOP specialists are actively involved in outreach efforts to increase program participation among those with the greatest barriers to employment.

Intensive Services provided by DVOP specialists include: assessments, employment plans, career guidance, referral to supportive services and training, connection to job openings.

Local Veteran Employment Representative (LVER): LVER staff conduct outreach to employers and engage in advocacy efforts with hiring executives to increase employment opportunities for veterans, encourage the hiring of disabled veterans and generally assist veterans to gain and retain employment. LVER staff conduct seminars for employers and job search workshops for veterans seeking employment, and facilitate priority of service in regard to employment, training, and placement services furnished to veterans by all staff of the employment service offices.

GOLD CARD PROGRAM

The Gold Card provides unemployed post-9/11 era veterans with the intensive and follow-up services they need to succeed in today's job market. The Gold Card initiative is a joint effort of the Department of Labor's Employment and Training Administration (ETA) and the Veterans' Employment and Training Service (VETS).

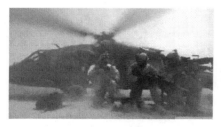

An eligible veteran can present the Gold Card at his/her local One-Stop Career Center to receive enhanced intensive services including up to six months of follow-up. The enhanced in-person services available for Gold Card holders at local One-Stop Career Center may include:

Job readiness assessment, including interviews and Testing-Development of an Individual Development Plan (IDP)

- Career guidance through group or individual counseling that helps veterans in making training and career decisions
- Provision of labor market, occupational, and skills transferability information that inform educational, training, and occupational decisions
- Referral to job banks, job portals, and job Openings-Referral to employers and registered apprenticeship sponsors
- Referral to training by WIA-funded or third-party service Providers-Monthly follow-up by an assigned case manager for up to six months

CIVILIAN CREDENTIALING ASSISTANCE

A product for Army and Navy Service members, Credentialing Opportunities On-Line (COOL) defines civilian credentials which best map to their Military Occupational Specialties, ratings, jobs, designators, and collateral duties/assignments. It outlines the path, work, training and experience required to achieve them. COOL also provides "how to" instructions for pursuing credentials, links to credentialing organizations, and cross-references to programs that may help Service members pay for credentialing fees.

U.S. ARMY WARRIOR TRANSITION COMMAND – EMPLOYER RESOURCES

When service members become wounded, ill, or injured, they often face a change in their career trajectory. While approximately 50% return to their military careers, many separate from service and begin a new career in the civilian workforce. These Veterans are well-trained, highly skilled professionals who can strengthen any organization, increasing diversity and the bottom line. There is no standard definition of a "wounded warrior" - today's military personnel experience a wide range of injuries, from amputations and burns to traumatic brain injury (TBI) and post-traumatic stress disorder (PTSD). What is most important is that these injuries do not prevent them from contributing to society, but often make them more resilient, determined, and ready to serve.

America's Heroes at Work is a U.S Department of Labor (DOL) project that addresses the employment challenges of returning Service Members and Veterans, especially those living with Traumatic Brain Injury (TBI) and/or Post-Traumatic-Stress-Disorder (PTSD)

VOW to Hire Heroes Act Tax Credit Information

The Work Opportunity Tax Credit (WOTC) is a Federal tax credit available to private sector businesses and certain non-profit organizations for hiring certain individuals, including veterans, who have consistently faced significant barriers to employment.

The WOTC program enables the targeted employees to gradually move from economic dependency into self-sufficiency as they earn a steady income, while participating employers are able to reduce their federal income tax liability.

TOP 10 REASONS TO HIRE VETERANS

Accelerated learning curve. Veterans have the proven ability to learn new skills and concepts. In addition, they can enter your workforce with identifiable and transferable skills, proven in real-world situations. This background can enhance your organization's productivity.

Leadership. The military trains people to lead by example as well as through direction, delegation, motivation, and inspiration. Veterans understand the practical ways to manage behaviors for results, even in the most trying circumstances. They also know the dynamics of leadership as part of both hierarchical and peer structures.

Teamwork. Veterans understand how genuine teamwork grows out of a responsibility to one's colleagues. Military duties involve a blend of individual and group productivity. They also necessitate a perception of how groups of all sizes relate to each other and an overarching objective.

Diversity and Inclusion in action. Veterans have learned to work side by side with individuals regardless of diverse race, gender, geographic origin, ethnic background, religion, and economic status as well as mental, physical, and attitudinal capabilities. They have the sensitivity to cooperate with many different types of individuals.

Efficient performance under pressure. Veterans understand the rigors of tight schedules and limited resources. They have developed the capacity to know how to accomplish priorities on time, in spite of tremendous stress. They know the critical importance of staying with a task until it is done right.

Respect for procedures. Veterans have gained a unique perspective on the value of accountability. They can grasp their place within an organizational framework, becoming responsible for subordinates' actions to higher supervisory levels. They know how policies and procedures enable an organization to exist.

Technology and Globalization. Because of their experiences in the service, veterans are usually aware of international and technical trends pertinent to business and industry. They can bring the kind of global outlook and technological savvy that all enterprises of any size need to succeed.

Integrity. Veterans know what it means to do "an honest day's work." Prospective employers can take advantage of a track record of integrity, often including security clearances. This integrity translates into qualities of sincerity and trustworthiness.

Conscious of health and safety standards. Thanks to extensive training, veterans are aware of health and safety protocols both for themselves and the welfare of others. Individually, they represent a drug-free workforce that is cognizant of maintaining personal health and fitness. On a company level, their awareness and conscientiousness translate into protection of employees, property, and materials.

Triumph over adversity. In addition to dealing positively with the typical issues of personal maturity, veterans have frequently triumphed over great adversity. They likely have proven their mettle in mission critical situations demanding endurance, stamina, and flexibility. They may have overcome personal disabilities through strength and determination.

A.R.S. 15-1802 - In-State Tuition for Honorably Discharged Veterans

Beginning in the fall semester of 2011, a person who is honorably discharged from the armed forces of the United States shall be granted immediate classification as an in-state student on honorable discharge from the Armed Forces and, while in continuous attendance toward the degree for which currently enrolled, does not lose in-state student classification if the person has met the following requirements:

1. Registered to vote in this state
2. Demonstrated objective evidence of intent to be a resident of Arizona that, for the purposes of this section, includes at least one of the following:

(a) An Arizona driver license.
(b) Arizona motor vehicle registration.
(c) Employment history in Arizona.
(d) Transfer of major banking services to Arizona.
(e) Change of permanent address on all pertinent records.
(f) Other materials of whatever kind or source relevant to domicile or residency status.

I AM AN AMERICAN SOLDIER

I AM A WARRIOR AND A MEMBER OF A TEAM

I SERVE THE PEOPLE OF THE UNITED STATES

I WILL ALWAYS PLACE THE MISSION FIRST

I WILL NEVER ACCEPT DEFEAT

I WILL NEVER QUIT

I WILL NEVER LEAVE A FALLEN COMRADE

I AM A GUARDIAN OF FREEDOM AND

THE AMERICAN WAY OF LIFE

I AM AN AMERICAN SOLDIER

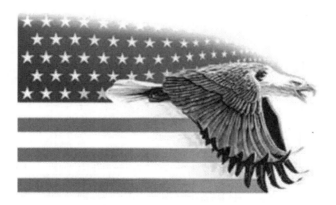

Arizona State Parks & Recreation Areas

"In war, there are no unwounded soldiers."
– Jose Narosky

Arizona State Parks protects and preserves 27 State Parks and Natural Areas. The agency also includes the State Trails Program, outdoor-related Grants Programs, the State Historic Preservation Office, as well as the Off-Highway Vehicle Program, and more. Arizona State Parks provides over 1,400 camping and RV sites throughout the state and manages 8 of the top 25 most visited natural attractions in Arizona. Selected parks now have online reservations.

Arizona State Parks Veterans Discount Program:

Active Duty Personnel, Guard and Reserves and state militia troops and up to three (3) accompanying adult family members receive 50% off the regular Day Use Fee to Arizona State Parks. *

A discount of 50% off day-use is available to all Arizona-resident (Arizona Driver's License address required) retired military Veterans and up to three (3) accompanying adult family members.

A 50% off discount is available to all Service-Disabled (10% - 90% or 100% Individual Unemployability), Veterans and up to three (3) accompanying adult family members. You must provide proof of military service and a verbal or written statement of your Service-Connected Disability.

A ***FREE*** day-use pass is available to all 100% Service-Connected Disabled Veterans and up to three (3) accompanying adult family members. You must provide a Veterans Administration-Certified letter of proof of your 100% Service-Connected Disability.

*The discount does not apply to Kartchner Caverns tour tickets, special-use fees, special program fees, special events fees, special event admission fees, any applicable reservation fees, camping fees or overnight parking fees at Arizona State Parks. You must present a military ID at park entrance to receive the discount.

The Arizona State Parks Department announced from the Fort Verde State Historic Park that the agency will be instituting a new program to provide Arizona's 100% permanently disabled veterans with a "Disabled Veterans Annual Day Use Pass". The pass will provide qualified veterans with day use access to all 27 State Parks.

For more information about Arizona State Parks or to get information on what each State Park has to offer, you can go to their website listed below or just give them a call at the number(s) listed.

Arizona State Parks
1300 West Washington Street
Phoenix, AZ 85007
Phone: (602)-542-4174
Toll Free: 1-800-285-3703
www.azstateparks.com

Travelers Information Service
Call 511 in Arizona
www.az511.gov

"This nation will remain the land of the free only so long as it is the home of the brave." – Elmer Davis

You will need to visit the website or call the number listed for each Ranger District to find out what the fees are (fees vary). The America the Beautiful Pass will get you up to 50% off the usage fees for most campgrounds. Discount Passes are not valid for Group sites, Double sites and on Cabin rentals. For more information on camping facilities, or to make your reservation, visit the website: www.recreation.gov.

Apache – Sitgreaves National Forest
30 South Chiricahua Drive
P.O. Box 640
Springerville, AZ 85938
Phone: 928-333-4301
www.fs.fed.us/r3/asnf

The Apache-Sitgreaves National Forest administered as one national forest, encompasses over two million acres of magnificent mountain country in east-central Arizona. Named after Captain Lorenzo Sitgreaves, a government topographical engineer who conducted the first scientific expedition across Arizona in the early 1850's.

What makes the forest so special? It's the water.... lots of it.... draining from the high mountains and forming numerous lakes and streams.... a fisherman's paradise in the arid Southwest.

The Apache-Sitgreaves National Forest has 34 lakes and reservoirs and more than 680 miles of rivers and streams – more than can be found in any other Southwestern National Forest. The White Mountains contain the headwaters of several Arizona Rivers including the Black, the Little Colorado and the San Francisco.

The major attractions for visitors from the desert are the Mollogon Rim and eight water lakes. From the Mollogon Rim's 7,600-foot elevation, vista points provide inspiring views of the low-lands to the south.

The Mollogon Rim (pronounced muggy-own) extends two hundred miles from Flagstaff into western New Mexico. The Apache-Sitgreaves National Forest ranges in elevation from 3,500 feet to nearly 11,500 feet. The area from Mount Baldy east to Escudilla Mountain is often referred to as the White Mountains of Arizona. From the edge of the Mollogon Rim, south of Hannagan Meadow, the land chops precipitously into the high desert around Clifton, Arizona.

For information on the various lodging and camping and fishing throughout this forest, contact the U.S. Forest Service at the website above or you can call them at the number(s) provided.

Coconino National Forest
1824 South Thompson Street
Flagstaff, AZ 86004
Phone: 928-527-3600
www.fs.fed.us/r3/coconino

Located in central Arizona, lies the Coconino National Forest. Northward lies the Colorado Plateau, a high, cold desert of flat-lying rocks and sheer-walled canyons. Southward lie hot desert basins and rugged mountains – the "basin and range province" which includes the Sonoran Desert of the southern Arizona. From the snow-frosted San Francisco Peaks to desert highlands along the Verde River, Coconino National Forest's 1.8 million acres drop 10,000 feet in elevation and cover a remarkable variety of landscapes.

Here you can climb the highest mountain in Arizona, fish in crystal-clear lakes, swim in the desert creeks under red rock cliffs and magnificent sycamore trees, float suspended under a hang glider from the crest of a cinder cone, or ski through parks and meadows and ponderosa pines.

The Coconino National Forest is one of the most diverse National Forests in the country with landscapes ranging from the famous red rocks of Sedona to Ponderosa Pine forests, from southwestern desert to alpine tundra. Explore mountains and canyons, fish in small lakes, and wade in lazy creeks and streams.

For information on the various lodging and camping and fishing throughout this forest, contact the U.S. Forest Service at the website above or you can call them at the number(s) provided.

Coronado National Forest

300 West Congress Street
Tucson, AZ 85701
Phone: 520-388-8300
www.fs.fed.us/r3/coronado

The Coronado National Forest welcomes you to its two southernmost ranger districts – Sierra Vista and Nogales – which include some of the most unusual mountain and range country in Arizona.

In an area, famous for brilliant sun and expansive desert, isolated mountains rise from the savannas. These peaks, nearly 9,000 feet above sea level, support forests, which offer relief from the lowland heat, as well as a wide range of recreational opportunities. They are ecological islands where distinct species of plants and animals have evolved.

Coronado National Forest: Sierra Vista and Nogales Ranger Districts provide information on recreational uses, local plants and wildlife, surface management, trails, roads, streams, lakes, visitor centers, facilities available, campgrounds, and picnic areas.

For information on the various lodging and camping and fishing throughout this forest, contact the U.S. Forest Service at the website above or you can call them at the number provided.

Kaibab National Forest

800 South 5th Street
Williams, AZ 86046
Phone: 928-635-8200
www.fs.fed.us/r3/kai

Located in northern Arizona, lies the Kaibab National Forest.
The Grand Canyon of the Colorado River divides the North Kaibab and Tusayan Ranger Districts of the Kaibab National Forest. Elevations within the forest are as low as 5,500 feet in the southwest to a high of 10,418 feet on Kendrick Mountain near the east boundary. Most of the terrain is relatively level, except for numerous small knolls, a few mountains, the Mollogon Rim that cuts diagonally across the southwest portion of the forest, and Coconino Rim on Tusayan Ranger District.

27

Pinon-Juniper woodlands are at lower elevations, Ponderosa pine forests are at middle elevations, and mixed conifer interspersed with aspen are at the highest elevations.

Camping on the Kaibab National Forest is limited to 14-days in any 30-day period. Developed campsites are available for a fee on a first-come, first-served basis; group sites, however, must be reserved in advance. Each campground has water faucets and toilets and each site has a picnic table and fire ring with grill. No electrical, sewage or water hookups are available at any of the campgrounds. A fee dump station is available at Kaibab Lake, Dogtown and Whitehorse Lake campgrounds. Campfires are restricted to existing fire rings or fire grates.

There are many undeveloped campsites and picnic spots in the forest. Visitors are welcome to use any of them but remember that camping is not permitted within ¼ mile of water, except in developed campgrounds. This helps protect the vegetation and the wildlife. Surface water in its natural condition may be unsafe to drink and should always be properly treated.

All streams located on the Williams Ranger District are intermittent and are not suitable for fishing. Fishing here occurs at lakes, many of which have developed campgrounds nearby. Some people do fish at a few of the larger tanks, including J.D. Dam, Perkins, Hells Canyon and Bar Cross Tanks. Due to the scarcity of navigational waters, only a limited amount of boating is done in the forest. If boating is permitted, only single gasoline engines with 8 horsepower or less are permitted on most lakes. Most boating is done in conjunction with fishing activities. Lake surface areas vary from about 40 to 70 acres.

They can accommodate small fishing boats, kayaks, canoes, and small (one- to two-person) sailboats or rafts.

For information on the various lodging and camping and fishing throughout this forest, contact the U.S. Forest Service at the website above or you can call them at the number provided

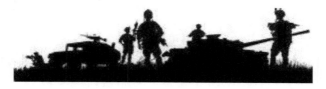

Prescott National Forest

344 Cortez Street
Prescott, AZ 86303-4398
Phone: 928-443-8094
Phone: 928-443-8000
Website: www.fs.fed.us/r3/prescott

The Forest is located about 70 air miles northwest of Phoenix, Arizona, contains approximately 1,237,000 acres, and is composed of two distinct divisions. The eastern portion of the Forest, which forms the headwaters of the Verde River, is bordered on the north by the Kaibab National Forest, on the east by the Coconino National Forest, and on the south by the Tonto National Forest. The western portion of the Forest, which includes the Bradshaw and Santa Maria Mountain ranges, is separated from the eastern portion by a broad patchwork of state, private, and other Federal lands. It forms the southern and western boundaries of the town of Prescott, the first capital of the territory of Arizona.

The forest contains 10 campgrounds, 4 group reservation campgrounds, 7 picnic areas, and 2 group reservation picnic areas. Most of the developed recreation sites are located in the pines with 5 of the campgrounds and two of the picnic areas situated near manmade lakes. Several developed sites offer barrier-free access for users experiencing disabilities.

Nearly 450 miles of scenic trails for hiking, backpacking, horseback riding, or mountain biking are offered on the Prescott National Forest.

The Forest also contains one National Recreational Trail (Granite Mountain Trail) and one National Historic Study Trail (General Crook Trail). The mild climate allows the trails to be enjoyed year-round.

For information on the various lodging and camping and fishing throughout this forest, contact the U.S. Forest Service at the website above or you can call them at the number provided.

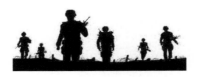

Tonto National Forest

2324 East Mc Dowell Road
Phoenix, AZ 85006
Phone: 602-225-5200
602-225-5395 TTY
602-236-5929
www.fs.fed.us/r3/tonto

Snuggled along the crest of the Mollogon Rim and stretching 90 miles south, the Tonto national Forest spreads over a spectacular 2.9 million acres of pine and cactus country just northwest of Phoenix, Arizona. To the north along the Rim country, cool, pine-covered slopes and clear trout-stocked streams attract thousands from the cities when summer temperatures soar. Just over the top of the Rim wooded lakes on the Coconino and Apache-Sitgreaves National Forests beckon hundreds more on weekends. When sun and sizzling urban asphalt push temperatures past the 100-degree mark, only the early birds find vacant Forest Service developed campgrounds.

Relief from desert heat inspires a great many people to travel to the cool waters of one of the six reservoirs on the Tonto National Forest. There is a considerable variation in the scenery, size, and type of opportunities found on these reservoirs.

Some people choose the larger lakes for water-skiing and power boating. While others opt for the quieter seclusion of a narrow lake arm extending between two near-vertical canyon walls. The Tonto National Forest has much to offer for boating enthusiasts. Enjoy your boating experience – but play it safe.

The Tonto National Forest has a collection of nearly 900 miles of National Forest System Trails. Their primary purpose is to provide a variety of opportunities for hikers, bikers and equestrians to enjoy the beauty and challenge of nature. The trail conditions range from good to very poor, most are not suitable for motor vehicles of any type. A trailing experience can include anything from the fulfilling opposition of steep grades and heavy brush, to the exciting discovery of spectacular scenic views and memorable and peaceful seclusion from the pressures and congestion of city life.

Exploring a trail in the Forest can be both relaxing and exhilarating, and sometimes even dangerous. With summer temperatures averaging in the mid 90's throughout most of the Forest, no trail adventures should be made without the appropriate precautionary measures. Make sure that you have an adequate supply of drinking water, as well as a general idea of the time needed to complete the trip.

It's also a good idea to take someone with you. You can run into trouble on any adventure, and sometimes the best defense is a partner or group. Remember to be safe when hiking and avoid unnecessary danger in all forms.

For information on the various lodging and camping and fishing throughout this forest, contact the U.S. Forest Service at the website above or you can call them at the number provided.

"The U. S. Military is us. There is no truer representation of a country than the people that it sends into the field to fight for it. The people who wear our uniform and carry our rifles into combat are our kids, and our job is to support them, because they're protecting us."
~Tom Clancy (1947-2013), author

Arizona Lakes and Water Recreation Areas

"People sleep peaceably in their beds at night only because rough men stand ready to do violence on their behalf." - George Orwell

Fishing and camping go together. There is nothing like pitching a tent in the pristine wilderness, on the edge of a lake or river, casting out a line and pulling in a rainbow trout, brook or brown trout – especially if the fish is later wrapped in foil and cooked over a roaring campfire.

Arizona's diverse topography and climate – from the Sonoran Desert in the southern part of the state to the mountains and canyons in the north – makes it a great place to set up camp and fish.

Camping at the lake adds fun activities like swimming, fishing, boating and water skiing to any camping trip. Arizona has many great lakes with camping areas or campgrounds near the lake. Pack up the tent and boat and take the family camping at one of these camping lakes soon. Some lakes in Arizona may require reservations to camp. If you plan to go fishing, local and/or state fishing licenses may be required. On some lakes canoe or boat rentals are available.

Arizona is blessed with diverse fishing opportunities, from the large reservoirs to the trout lakes in the mountains, and plenty of low-elevation fishing holes in between. Go out and catch yourself a memory!

Many of the lakes contain game fish and are managed by the Arizona Game and Fish Department. Some lakes may dry out or freeze out fish and will require seasonal restocking. Most lakes will not allow large motorboats.

Due to Arizona's dry climate, many of the lakes listed here are intermittent lakes and do not contain water throughout the entire year.

There are 128 lakes, reservoirs, ponds, and marshes in Arizona. You can find out more about these bodies of water and what varieties of fish species are stocked and what discounts are available for Military and Veterans in Arizona, by contacting the Arizona Game and Fish Department at http://www.azgfd.gov.

HUNTING AND FISHING PRIVILEGES

Resident hunting and fishing licenses for members of the Armed Forces on active duty, stationed in state are available upon application. Complimentary licenses may be granted to veterans 70 years or older who have been residing in Arizona for at least 25 years. Complimentary licenses will be issued to veterans that are verified by the U.S. Department of Veterans Affairs to be 100% service–connected disabled and who have been a resident for one year or more.

If you need information about the various campgrounds and camping areas and what they have to offer and any fees, you can contact the United States Forest Service at www.fs.fed.us

Arizona Ski Areas

"The soldier is the army. No army is better than its soldiers. The Soldier is also a citizen. In fact, the highest obligation and privilege of citizenship is that of bearing arms for one's country."

— Gen. George S. Patton

Mention Arizona and most people who have never been here before conjuring up images of hot arid desert and cactus. But Arizona also has forested mountain peaks and deep ski bases topped with powdered snow perfect for snow skiing during the winter months in the higher elevation areas. All Arizona ski areas feature slopes for all skill levels including beginners, young children and advanced skiers.

Arizona Snowbowl Ski Resort & Summer Scenic Skyride

9300 N. Snowbowl Rd.
Flagstaff, AZ 86001
Phone: (928)-779-1951
(928)-774-0729 or 1-800-472-3599 (in CA and AZ only) - lodging and reservations
www.arizonasnowbowl.com
SkiLiftLodge@arizonasnowbowl.com

Arizona Snowbowl Ski Lift Lodge & Cabins

6355 North Highway 180
Flagstaff, AZ 86001
928-774-0729

Considered by many to be the premier Arizona ski resort, Snowbowl is just 15 miles from Flagstaff in the majestic San Francisco Peaks. With five lifts serving 32 runs ranging from easy to difficult, Snowbowl has a base elevation of 9,200 feet with the summit soaring to over 11,000 feet above the lush valley below.

One impressive trail boasts a 2,300-foot vertical drop and the entire Snowbowl Mountain covers 777 ski-able acres, making the Arizona Snowbowl one of the largest and most challenging ski areas in the West.

Open to both skiers and snowboarders, Snowbowl also boasts a Terrain Park with rails and spines that sharpen the skills of even the most expert boarders. Two mountain day lodges nearby are open with restaurants and lounges for that midday break, and the Snowbowl has a premier equipment rental shop and ski school with instructors for every level. Families will appreciate the special instruction programs for children, while even the best skiers can drop in for a quick tune-up on their techniques.

Arizona Snowbowl is 2 hours from Phoenix, and 70 miles from the Grand Canyon. The resort opened in 1938 and is now one of the oldest continually operated ski area in the country.

Once you reach Flagstaff, I-17 becomes Milton Road. Continue driving north for 3 miles. Milton Road will go under the railroad tracks and the road will bear to the right. Take a left at the first stop light (Humphreys Street). At the third stop light (Hwy 180), turn left. Continue 7 miles to Snowbowl Road and then turn right (just past mile marker 222). The resort is 7 miles up Snowbowl Road.

WAYS TO SAVE AT SNOWBOWL

- **25% OFF** regular admission when you purchase your tickets online
- **50% OFF** regular admission for groups of 10 or more guests with at least a 48-hour reservation
- **FREE** ticket on your birthday! Present a valid ID at the counter to receive your complimentary ticket
- **FREE** ticket with your 2012-13 Winter Season Pass. Present your pass at the ticket counter and receive your FREE Skyride ticket
- **All military** (active duty, retired, reserve and dependents) **receive 25% OFF Skyride tickets.** Must present valid Military ID.

Snowbowl does offer an adaptive skiing program. It is $50 for a 3-hour lesson, including lift ticket or $100 for a 6-hour lesson, including lift ticket. A two-week advanced notice is required so that they can plan the best experience possible.

Flagstaff Nordic Center

US 180-Coconino Forest 86002
928-220-0550
www.flagstaffnordiccenter.com

Tucked into the San Francisco Peaks in the Coconino National Forest about 15 miles from downtown Flagstaff, this Nordic oasis has most of the common attributes one would associate with a good cross country ski center anywhere else in the country. Flagstaff Nordic Center has a full 40km of non-redundant trails, more if you count portions of trails that you have to repeat to reach more distant loops.

The trails wind through some of the largest Ponderosa pine stands in the state with the ever-present aspen, the other dominant species. Trails are named for terrain features found throughout the region, most of which are named after significant individuals and historic figures.

We are the perfect base camp for your winter adventures in the Southwest! Enjoy staying in one of our large or small yurts or a log-sided camper cabin in the foothills of the San Francisco Peaks! During the summer season, we are now offering mountain bike tours and rentals! Enjoy the peace and quiet of the Coconino National Forest. Explore over 50 km of well-marked trails by bike or foot. Wildlife is abundant as most areas of the center are designated No Motorized Vehicles by the United States Forest Service. During the winter season enjoy the well-groomed cross-country ski trails of Flagstaff Nordic Center. We offer over 40 km of ski trails groomed for both classic and skate style skiing. With over 15 km of well-marked snowshoe trails we are the perfect location for a winter hike.

Winter Season: Mid-December through March (if there's snow)

Hours: 9:00 a.m.-4:30 p.m. daily.

Summer Season: May through October

Location: 16 miles north of Flagstaff on paved and plowed roads. Elevation is 8,000 feet.

Drive 16 miles north from Flagstaff on US 180 and look for the Flagstaff Nordic Center signs at mile marker 232.

Elk Ridge Ski and Outdoor Recreation Area

2467 South Perkinsville Road
Williams, AZ 86046
928-814-5038
www.elkridge.com
Email: info@elkridgeski.com

Although the name has changed, you can be sure that Elk Ridge Ski Area in historic Williams, Arizona is the same family friendly ski resort that has operated for years as the Williams Ski Area. Although the area is the smallest of the four ski areas in Arizona, it has 37 ski-able acres for skiing, snowboarding for those of differing abilities. Elk Ridge considers itself a family mountain both with its employees and with their customers. Being a small ski area, there are no lift lines or crowds, with wonderful variety of terrain and great people. In addition, the varied terrain of this resort offers year-round tubing. and offers skiing, snowboarding and tubing for all ages. Located at the southern gateway to the Grand Canyon South Rim just minutes from downtown Williams, Elk Ridge Ski Area boasts a newly renovated day lodge, snack bar, poma lift and beginners slope area, all run by friendly staffers who's number one goal is to make sure you have fun in the snow.

The resort is located 30 miles west of Flagstaff, Arizona, in the town of Williams, Arizona, and the "Gateway to the Grand Canyon." From Highway 40, once you have arrived in the historic town of Williams, drive south on 4th street (becomes Perkinsville Road); approximately 2.5 miles to Ski Run Road (also posted as Forest Service Road 106), the sign is on the right, take Ski Run Road 1.5 miles to Elk Ridge.

Open Thursday through Monday during the season, starting mid-December. traditionalists will love the Skiers Only Thursdays while snowboarders and the tube enthusiasts find the short lines and small crowds perfect for weekend trips. The ski shop offers Elan equipment for rent and quality instructors on hand for those looking to improve their skills on the slopes.

Priding itself on family fun, Elk Ridge Ski Area has a newly groomed tube hill and all new tubes, making for a safe gliding experience for everyone in the family. There are even family discounts available and kids age 4 and under are free with a paid adult.

Come visit for skiing, snowboarding and tubing during the winter months. Soon they will add new services like horseback riding, guided tours and Grand Canyon packages!

Lodge facilities include equipment rentals, both skiing and snowboarding lessons. There is a snack bar service. The lodge is also home to First Aid services by National Ski Patrol.

Mount Lemmon Ski Valley

10300 Ski Run Rd
Mt. Lemmon, AZ 85619
520-576-1321
www.skithelemmon.com
Email: graham@skithelemmon.com

During World War II, a group of skiers made up of Lowell Thomas, a noted journalist and adventurer, a local forest ranger, and many Davis Monthan servicemen that included Thomas' son, later a Governor of Alaska, and Art Devlin, a future Olympic ski jumper and Television commentator, formed the Saguaro Ski Club. The well - known cartoonist, Paul Webb, created a patch and membership certificates for the club showing a skier wrapped around a saguaro cactus. Thomas sent honorary memberships to dozens of friends, famous personalities around the world, making membership a tongue in cheek must. A ski gala was held that first year at the Arizona Inn with many of Thomas' friends in attendance.

A Forest Service lease was obtained, an old model "A" with its tires removed propelled a rope tow and Mt. Lemmon Ski Valley had its beginning.

Few people think of snow and skiing when they think of Tucson, AZ. Mount Lemmon Ski Valley is located on the slopes of Mount Lemmon in the Santa Catalina Mountains just north of Tucson, Arizona. It is part of the Coronado national Forest, located near the mountaintop village of Summerhaven. The summit is 9,157 feet above sea level and receives approximately 180 inches of snow annually. Located in Mt. Lemmon, Arizona, with 21 ski trails served by 3 lifts. Located just an hour's drive from the sun-drenched resorts of Tucson, area visitors can go golfing, swimming and downhill skiing in the same day.

With a ski area covering over 200 acres and an annual snowfall reaching over 200 inches, Mt. Lemmon offers trails for every ski level, with 20% of runs considered perfect for beginners and 38% just slightly more difficult. Expert skiers should not be discouraged; however, Mt. Lemmon is home to several "Expert Only" trails as well, making the area the perfect ski experience for everyone. In need of extra equipment or want to improve your technique with a lesson or two?

Lemmon Ski valley also has premiere equipment rentals and top-notch instructors on hand to meet all your ski-related needs.

Winter storms on Mount Lemmon are frequent, leaving untouched powder areas. The ski season on Mount Lemmon usually occurs between mid-December and April. The weather is usually mild enough to ski in a sweater and denim jeans, with temperatures ranging from 20 to 50 degrees Fahrenheit. There no grooming at Mt. Lemmon, which makes even the mild terrain challenging. Ski Valley is accessible via the Catalina Highway. Parking is limited at the ski area.

The ski lift runs year-round, as a "Sky Ride" experience in the summertime, offering views of the Ski Valley area, forest and grass-covered slopes, and the long-distance vistas of the mountains and valleys in the distance north of the Santa Catalina's, the city of Tucson, the San Pedro Valley, the Reef of Rocks, and the distant mountains near Globe and Phoenix.

Mount Lemmon is open daily from 9 A.M. to 4 P.M. Half-day starts at 12:30 P.M.

Mount Lemmon offers a discount for active duty ONLY. They do not have a "written" plan for an adaptive ski program, but if you are disabled and would like to ski, the rental and ski personnel can make something happen. ***So, come enjoy the slopes and SKI!***

Sunrise Park Resort

Highway 273 Greer
Pinetop-Lakeside, AZ 85927
928--735-7669
1-800-772-7669
www.sunriseskipark.com

Sunrise Park Resort is a ski resort located near Greer, close to the border of New Mexico. The resort consists of three mountains named Sunrise Peak, Cyclone Peak and Apache Peak. Situated on the Colorado Plateau and perched atop the White Mountains in eastern Arizona, with a base of 9,200 feet and spread across three peaks and 800 acres, Sunrise tops out at 11,100 feet above sea level at Apache Peak. Sunrise offers 65 runs of varying terrain, promising a great ski experience for everyone. Families with children will enjoy the Resort's "ski-wee" area while world-class downhill racers can access multiple runs each day on the Sunrise Express High Speed Quadlift. Snowboarders can find implanted rails and a snow half pipe in the Terrain Park and the whole family will enjoy sliding down the mountain inner-tube style.

Afterwards, cap off your day in the snow by taking an exciting sleigh ride through the woods or enjoy the Resort's indoor swimming pool and spa or just kick back and unwind by the fireplace or in one of the hotel's 100 relaxing rooms overlooking the spectacular mountain landscape.

The Resort is owned by the White Mountain Apache Tribe and is located on the Fort Apache Indian Reservation. The resort is a year-round recreation destination and offers a wide range of outdoor activities. During the winter, the resort's three mountains offer excellent alpine skiing. There are plenty of challenging runs for experienced skiers and an abundance of enjoyable intermediate runs for the not-so experienced skier. When Arizona experiences wet winters, which aren't too uncommon, Sunrise provides as good of skiing as anywhere in the Southwest. The ski season usually runs from December through March. Night skiing is occasionally offered in mid-January and mid-February. There is also a snowboard terrain park and separate cross-country skiing area.

The Sunrise Ski School offers personal, specialized instruction for skiers of all levels and ages. Their professional instructors have the experience to enhance your skills. Most of all, they know how to make you feel comfortable on terrain that is suited to your ability. Ski and Snowboard lessons are on a first come first served basis. Adult and junior group lessons begin at 10:00 am. Half-day lessons are 90 minutes of instruction. They also have available full-day lessons. Private lessons are available for both Adults and juniors. Sunrise offers a 10% discount for military and they offer adaptive skiing programs for their disabled customers.

For more information about Ski and Snowboard lessons, please contact the Ski School directly at 928-735-7669, Ext.#2306 or skischool@sunriseskipark.com -- please include your phone number for a faster reply.

Arizona Amusement Parks

"America without Her Soldiers would be like God without His angels."

- Claudia Pemberton

A girl on a surfboard in an Arizona water park, pool water parks, game rooms, train rides, rock-climbing walls, go-kart racing, and much, much more for kids of all ages and adults who still think they are kids. These amusement venues are great for family fun outings and birthday parties. Just bring a valid military ID card and ask for any discounts.

Amazing Jakes — Amazing Jake's is the first facility of its kind to open in the Phoenix area. Amazing Jake's is over 90,000 square feet of food and fun. We offer an all-indoor facility with the best buffet in town and the perfect location for your Birthday Parties, Group Events, Corporate Outings, or to spend some quality time with family and friends.

Amazing Jake's features an Amazing All-U-Can-Eat Buffet with delicious Pizzas, Pastas, Soups, a Potato and Salad Bar with Unlimited Beverages and Desserts.

The Fun Factory includes over 150 Interactive Redemption and Video Games along with the biggest and best prize counter in town. Amazing Jake's also contains an Indoor Go-Kart track, a Glow Bowling Alley, Bumper Cars, a Mini Coaster and a brand-new attraction coming soon! We offer four kiddie rides including the Rio Grande Train, Tea Cups, a Frog Hopper as well as a Carousel. www.amazingjakes.com

Alltel Ice Den — In Scottsdale, it is a 150,000-square foot, state-of-the-art, twin ice-skating and entertainment facility and still home of the Phoenix Coyotes Hockey Team. Also, within the facility, is the Mountainside Fitness Training Center and the Over Easy Breakfast Diner and 18 Degrees, North Scottsdale's newest neighborhood grill. www.coyoteice.com

Big Surf – Located in Tempe. A full mix of rides for the entire family. Challenge Hurricane Falls, a thrilling speed slide. Captain Cook's Landing will enthrall your little ones. Is America's original wavepool, with over 2 million gallons of water. Big Surf offers active duty military, police, fire discounts. Free admission on Armed Forces Day. www.bigsurffun.com

Breakers Waterpark – In Marana. Arizona's largest wavepool with 1.3 million gallons of wavepool excitement! Enjoy the morning with your children at the new Captain Kidd's Surfari. www.breakerswaterpark.com

Castle's and Coaster's – In Phoenix. Whether you are young or old, big or small, you will find lots of fun, food, and excitement at Arizona's Finest Fun and Thrill Park. $5.00 off regular prices for our active duty and retired customers. Disabled customers can go to the front of each line along with a reasonable number of guests. www.castlesandcoasters.com

Cracker Jax Family Fun – In Scottsdale. Cracker Jax is Arizona's largest family fun and Sports Park with over 27 acres of excitement! www.crackerjax.com

Desert Breeze Railroad Park – In Chandler. Fun starts right away at the old-time train station. Enjoy rides, a lake and playground area. Great birthday party venue! www.desertbreezerr.com

Enchanted Island Amusement Park – In Phoenix. Filled with charm and magic, offering nine fanciful rides and a variety of popular attractions geared especially toward children ages 2 to 10. www.enchantedisland.com

F-1 Race Factory – In Phoenix. America's largest indoor kart racing and entertainment venue. Everything from high-speed European kart racing to rock climbing, billiards and a wide selection of arcade games. www.octaneraceway.com

Funtasticks – In Tucson. Offers mini-golf, go-karts, bumper boats, a 5-ride Kiddie Land, and a state-of-the-art video arcade with all-new games recently added. www.funtasticks.com

Freestone Park Railroad – In Gilbert. The park is home to softball fields, basketball courts, sand volleyball courts, batting cages, soccer fields, a skateboard park, and walking trails around 2 lakes that house several well-fed waterfowl. www.freestonerr.com

Golf & Stuff! – In Tucson. Golf & Stuff! Is proud to announce the arrival of their brand-new bumper boats! All new electric boats with super squirt guns so you can soak your friends. www.golfnstuff.com

Golfland SunSplash Waterpark – In Mesa. Experience the Master Blaster, a water roller coaster: tube uphill, rip down the other side and back up again! Challenge the Sidewinder half pipe thrill slide; a steep vertical drop sends you flying down first wall to the bottom. www.golfland.com

Jambo! – In Mesa. Designed to please children ages 2 to twelve. Jambo! is the ultimate family entertainment experience combining the rides and excitement of an outdoor amusement park. www.jambopark.com

McCormick-Stillman Railroad Park – In Scottsdale. Take a ride on the Paradise and Pacific Railroad and antique carousel. Visit a variety of shops and museum or play in one of the spacious playgrounds, or just relax in the grass under a tree or in one the park's picnic armadas. www.therailroadpark.com

He would be the first to answer the call
He would be the one who would give his all
He was first to stand up for what is right
He would help a stranger as well as a friend
He would offer his support until the end
He would give help to anyone in need
He would smile and always be in the lead
He would be the first to reach out his hand
He left his youth, signed up to go to war
He said it was his duty, held up his hand and swore
His oath to preserve and protect at any price
He did it willingly, without thinking twice
He paid the price of freedom by giving his life
He left behind a grieving family, a child and wife
His absence is a wound that can't be healed
His place in their lives will never be filled
He laid down his life for you and for me
He sacrificed his future so we could be free
He paid the debt that can never be repaid

- Kathryn Taylor

"Live for something rather than die for nothing. "

– Gen. George S. Patton

AMERICA THE BEAUTIFUL PASS

The National Parks and Federal Recreational Lands Pass

A pass is your ticket to more than 2,000 federal recreation sites. Each pass covers entrance fees at national parks and national wildlife refuges as well as standard amenity fees at national forests and grasslands, and at lands managed by the Bureau of Land management and the Bureau of Reclamation. A pass covers entrance and standard amenity fees for the driver and all passengers in a personal vehicle at per vehicle fee areas (up to four adults at sites that charge per person). Children age 15 and under are admitted free.

Annual Pass

- $80.00
- Available to everyone
- Can be obtained in person at a federal recreation site, or by calling 1-888-ASK USGS (1-888-275-8747), ext. #1, or online at www.nps.gov
- Non-transferable
- Free Annual Pass for U.S. Military
- Available to U.S. Military members and dependents in all branches of the Armed Forces.
- Must be obtained in person at a federal recreation site by showing a Military ID Card (Form 1173), or a CAC Card.

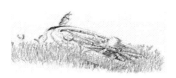

Senior Pass

- $10.00 Lifetime Pass
- For U.S. citizens or permanent residents age 62 or over
- May be obtained in person at a federal recreation site or through the mail, using the application form at www.nps.gov. Enter passes in Search. Then Click on U.S. National Park Service America the Beautiful. The cost of obtaining a Senior Pass through the mail is $20.00. ($10.00 for the Senior Pass and $10.00 for processing the application). Applicants must provide documentation of age and residency or citizenship.
- May provide a 50% discount on some amenity fees charged for facilities and services, such as camping, swimming, boat launch, and specialized interpretive services.
- Generally, does not cover or reduce special recreation permit fees or fees charged by concessionaires.

Access Pass

- Free
- For U.S. citizens or permanent residents with permanent disabilities.
- May be obtained in person at any BLM, FWS, NPS, Reclamation, and USDA-FS recreation fee areas, or through the mail using the application form at www.nps.gov. Enter passes in Search. Then Click on U.S.

National Park Service America the Beautiful Pass. The cost of obtaining an Access Pass through the mail is $10.00; for processing the application (the Pass is free). Applicants must provide documentation of permanent disability and residency or citizenship.

- Admits the pass holder and any accompanying passengers in a private vehicle. * for areas that charge a per person fee. * The pass admits the pass holder and 3 additional passengers (16 years and older). May provide a 50% discount on some amenity fees charged for facilities and services, such as camping, swimming, boat launch, and specialized interpretive services.

- Generally, does not cover or reduce special recreation permit fees or fees charged by concessionaires.

Volunteer Pass

- Free
- For volunteers with 250 service hours with federal agencies that participate in the Interagency Pass Program.
- Contact your local federal recreation site for more information about volunteer opportunities or visit: www.vounteer.gov

NOTE: Golden Access and Golden Age Passports are no longer sold. However, these passes will still be honored per the provisions of the pass.

Grand Canyon National Park

U.S. Department of Interior
National Park Service

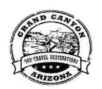

Address:
Grand Canyon National Park
P.O. Box 129
Grand Canyon, AZ 85023

Phone: 928-638-7888
E –mail: grca_information@nps.gov
Website: www.nps.gov/grcca

Elevation: South Rim – 7000 feet
North Rim – 8,000–9,000 feet
Phantom Ranch – 2,550 feet

High altitude sickness and other issues caused by elevation have the following symptoms:

- ❖ Shortness of breath
- ❖ Light-headedness
- ❖ Nausea and vomiting
- ❖ Headaches

North Rim Visitor Center
8 A.M. – 6 P.M. (9 A.M. – 4 P.M. after October 15th)

Mather Point

Wheelchair accessible with view of Colorado River and South Kaibab Trail Scenic Drive Accessibility Permit Available at entrance stations, in-park hotels, and visitor centers. For visitors with mobility issues.

Must be displayed on vehicle dashboard Allows personal vehicles on Hermit and Yaki Point roads. Does not qualify vehicles to park in designated handicap parking spaces

Trail of Time

Wheelchair accessible 1.3-mile (2.2 KM) trail between Verkamp's Visitor Center and Yavapai Geology Museum Touchable samples of Grand Canyon's rocks

Hermits Rest

Designed by Mary Colter and opened in 1914
Wheelchair accessible restrooms, snack bar, and gift shop

Tusayan Museum and Ruins

Learn about Traditionally Associated Tribes
Tour ancestral Puebloan village on wheelchair accessible trail.

Park Rangers are available to answer questions and describe exhibits.

Weather*

Summer: **Daytime average temperatures**
North and South Rims: 70–80's (21–32°C)
Inner Canyon: 100's (38–43°C)

Nighttime average temperatures
North and South Rims: 40–50's (4–15°C)
Inner Canyon: 70's (21–27°C)

*Monsoon rain during July to early September with dangerous lightning.

Winter: **Daytime average temperatures**
North and South Rims: 30–40's (-1–10°C)
Inner Canyon: 50–60's (10–21°C)

Nighttime average temperatures
North and South Rims: 10's (-12–7°C)
Inner Canyon: high 30's (2–4°C)

*Snow and ice

This information is current as of summer, 2015. For up-to-date information, see "The Guide", available at entrance stations, visitor centers, or visit www.nps.gov/grca.

Service Animals

Service animals are allowed in all facilities and on all shuttle buses and trails but must always be leashed. Persons wishing to take a service animal below the rim must first check in at the Backcountry Information Center.

Medical Facilities

Dial 911 in an emergency (9-911 from the in-park hotel rooms)
South Rim: North Country Clinic: (928)-638-2551
North Rim: There are no medical facilities; EMT's are available

Wheelchairs:

South Rim: Wheelchairs are available to rent at   Bright Angel Bicycles next to Grand Canyon Visitor Center. (928)-814-8704
North Rim: A limited number of wheelchairs are available for loan from the Visitor center, free of charge.

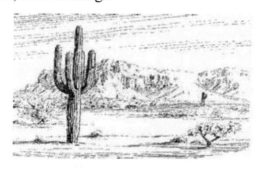

Petrified Forest National Park

Mailing Address:
1 Park Road, PO Box 2217
Petrified Forest, AZ 86028

Phone: 928-524-6228
Website: www.nps.gov/pefo/index.htm

Imagine walking back through time in a place where dinosaurs once roamed over 225 million years ago. A time when lush green forests ruled the landscape with 200-foot tall conifers. Volcanic mountains erupted toppling the trees, then they were swept away by waterways and covered with volcanic ash and sediment, these trees became entombed and over millions of years became petrified. Through gradual erosion, gigantic logs and remnant pieces became exposed for the world to experience.

The Petrified Forest is home to some of the most impressive fossils ever found. Fossils found here show that the Forest was once a tropical region, filled with towering trees and extraordinary creatures we can only begin to imagine. While more than 150 different species of fossilized plants have been discovered by paleontologists, species of reptiles, such as the Desmatosuchus, similar to the armadillo, have also been discovered.

Archaeologists have found much evidence to indicate that ancient native people inhabited this region about 10,000 years ago. Petroglyph drawings on rock surfaces, gives a glimpse of the past and you can see the marks of a solar calendar at Puerco Pueblo near the time of the summer solstice.

The Petrified Forest National Park is located in Navajo and Apache counties in northeastern Arizona. The park covers about 170 square miles, encompassing semi-desert shrub steppe as well as highly eroded and colorful badlands. The park, the northern part of which extends into the Painted Desert, was declared a national monument in 1906 and a national park in 1962.

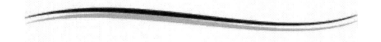

About 800,000 people visit the park each year and take part in activities including sightseeing, photography, hiking, and backpacking.

So, come for the adventure and discover what the Petrified Forest National Park has to offer!

Saguaro National Park

Address:
3693 South Old Spanish Trail
Tucson, AZ 85730

Phone: 520-733-5153
Website: www.nps.gov/sugu/htm

Think Arizona and the statuesque Saguaro Cactus usually comes to mind. It stands tall as an iconic symbol of Arizona as they seem to hold secrets to the days of the Old West. That's because many of these stately plants are thousands of years-old and were there to witness ancient Native American civilizations, the arrival of Spanish Explorers in the 1600s, the wagon trains of early American settlers and the "rough and tough" days of cowboys and outlaws.

Tucson, Arizona is home to the nation's largest cacti. The giant saguaro is the universal symbol of the American southwest. These majestic plants, found only in a small portion of the United States, are protected by the Saguaro National Park.

Here you have a chance to see these enormous cacti, silhouetted by the beauty of a magnificent desert sunset.

Saguaro National Park is located in southern Arizona on the outskirts of Tucson and is a part of the United States National Park System. The park has two districts - the Rincon Mountain District is located to the east of Tucson and rises to over 8,000 feet and includes over 128 miles of trails and the Tucson Mountain District which is located to the west of Tucson and is generally lower in elevation with a denser saguaro forest. The park preserves the desert landscape, fauna and flora contained within two park sections. The park was established to protect its namesake—the giant saguaro cactus and in 1933, the Saguaro National Monument was created. The Saguaro Wilderness

Area of 71,400 acres was added in 1975. Saguaro National Park was created from these areas in 1994 and currently encompasses 91,327 acres in its two districts. Saguaro in this park are near the northernmost limit of their natural survival zone within the Sonoran Desert.

Monument Valley Navaho Tribal Park

Mailing Address:
P.O. Box 7717
Shonto, AZ 86045

Phone: 928-672-2700 - Navajo National Monument Visitor Center Office Contact
Website: www.nps.gov/nava/index.htm

This great valley boasts sandstone masterpieces that tower at heights of 400 to 1,000 feet. framed by scenic clouds casting shadows that graciously roam the desert floor.

The angle of the sun accents these graceful formations, providing scenery that is simply spellbinding. The fragile pinnacles of rock are surrounded by miles of mesas and buttes, shrubs, trees and windblown sand and all of this comprising the magnificent colors of the valley.

Before human existence, the Park was once a vast lowland basin. For hundreds of millions of years, materials that eroded from the early Rock Mountains deposited layer upon layer of sediments which cemented a slow and gentle uplift generated by ceaseless pressure from below the surface, elevating these horizontal strata quite uniformly one to three miles above sea level. What was once a basin, became a plateau.

Natural forces of wind and water that eroded the land and spent the last 50 million years cutting in to and peeling away at the surface of the plateau.

The simple wearing down of altering layers of soft and hard rock slowly revealed the natural wonders of Monument Valley today.

From the visitor center, you see the world-famous panorama of the Mitten buttes and Merrick Butte. You can also purchase guided tours from Navajo tour operators, who will take you down into the valley in jeeps for a narrated cruise through these mythical formations. Places such as Ear of the Wind and other landmarks can only be accessed via guided tours.

During the summer months, the visitor center also features the Haskenneini Restaurant, which specializes in both native Navajo and American cuisines, and has a film/snack/souvenir shop as well. There are year-round restroom facilities.

One mile before the center, numerous Navajo vendors sell arts, crafts, native food and souvenirs at roadside stands.

Meteor Crater National Landmark

Address:
Meteor Crater Enterprises, Inc.
Interstate 40, Exit 233
Winslow, AZ 86047

Phone: 928-289-2362
Toll Free : 1-800-289-5898
Website: www.metyeorcrater.com
Email: info@meteorcrater.com

Meteor Crater is the breath-taking result of a collision between an asteroid traveling 26,000 miles per hour and planet Earth approximately 50,000 years ago. The Crater is nearly one mile across, 2.4 miles in circumference and more than 550 feet deep. It is an international tourist venue with outdoor observation trails, air-conditioned indoor viewing, wide screen movie theater, Interactive Discovery Center, unique gift and rock shop, and Astronaut Memorial Park at the Visitor Center located on the crater rim.

Because the United States Board on Geographic Names commonly recognizes names of natural features derived from the nearest post office, the feature acquired the name of "Meteor Crater" from the nearby post office named Meteor. The site was formerly known as the Canyon Diablo Crater and fragments of the meteorite are officially called the Canyon Diablo Meteorite. Scientists refer to the crater as Barringer Crater in honor of Daniel Barringer, who was first to suggest that it was produced by meteorite impact.

The crater is privately owned by the Barringer family through their Barringer Crater Company, which proclaims it to be the "best preserved meteorite crater on Earth".

Located approximately 37 miles east of Flagstaff and 18 miles west of Winslow in the northern Arizona desert.

Canyon de Chelly National Monument

Mailing Address:
P.O. Box 588
Chinle, AZ 86503

Phone: 928-674-5500
Website: www.nps.gov/cach/index.htm

Canyon de Chelly National Monument was established on April 1, 1931 as a unit of the National Park Service. It is located in northeastern Arizona within the boundaries of the Navajo Nation. Reflecting one of the longest continuously inhabited landscapes of North America, it preserves ruins of the early indigenous tribes that lived in the area, including the Ancient Pueblo Peoples and Navajo. The monument covers 83,840 acres and encompasses the floors and rims of the three major canyons: de Chelly, del Muerto, and Monument. These canyons were cut by streams with headwaters in the Chuska mountains just to the east of the monument. None of the land is federally owned. In 2009, Canyon de Chelly National Monument was recognized as one of the most-visited national monuments in the United States.

For nearly 5,000 years, people have lived in these canyons - longer than anyone has lived uninterrupted anywhere on the Colorado Plateau. In the place called Tseyi, their homes and images tell us their stories. Today, Navajo families make their homes, raise livestock, and farm the lands in these canyons. The National Park Service and Navajo Nation actively work together to manage park resources.

Beyond the Painted Desert, much of the far northeast of Arizona is barren and not particularly scenic, as the land-forms wide, empty valleys interspersed by low, scrub-covered mesas. Three of these, named the First, Second and Third, lie at the center of Hopi Indian territory but most of the northeast is Navajo land, including Chinle which is the largest town in the area and the gateway to Canyon de Chelly National Monument. This comparatively little-known canyon is not as immediately spectacular as others in Arizona or Utah but it does have sheer sandstone walls rising up to 1,000 feet, several scenic overlooks and many well-preserved Anasazi ruins, and the area provides a fascinating insight into the present-day life of the Navajo, who still inhabit and cultivate the valley floor.

Vermilion Cliffs National Monument

Address:
345 E. Riverside Drive
St. George, UT 84790-6714

Phone: 435-688-3200
Website:
www.blm.gov/az/st/en/prog/blm_special_areas/natmon/vermilion.html

In far north Arizona, just south of the Utah state line, is Vermilion Cliffs National Monument, a veritable natural treasure of astounding geology comprised of 293,689 acres of breathtaking Arizona beauty that protects the Paria Plateau, Vermilion Cliffs, Coyote Buttes, and Paria Canyon. This spectacular place is the most visible natural feature in one of five BLM-administered national monuments that were established in 2000. Like the other four,

Vermilion Cliffs National Monument is marked only by a few signposts and is likely to remain largely without any particular visitor facilities or other improvements - this is a place for people to explore by themselves, though still most tourists zip by on US 89 or US 89A, en-route between Zion National Park, the Grand Canyon and Lake Powell, without stopping in this scenic region.

Wupatki National Monument

Mailing Address:
6400 U.S. 89
Flagstaff, AZ 86004

Phone: 928-679-2365
Website: www.nps.gov/wupa/index.htm

Nestled between the Painted Desert and ponderosa highlands of northern Arizona, Wupatki is a landscape of legacies. Ancient pueblos dot red-rock outcroppings across miles of prairie. Where food and water seem impossible to find, people-built pueblos, raised families, farmed, traded, and thrived. Today, if you linger and listen, earth and artifacts whisper their stories to us still.

The Wupatki National Monument is a U.S. National Monument located in north-central Arizona, near Flagstaff. Rich in Native American ruins, the monument is administered by the National Park Service in close conjunction with the nearby Sunset Crater Volcano National Monument.

For its time and place, there was no other pueblo like Wupatki. Less than 800 years ago, it was the tallest, largest, and perhaps the richest and most influential pueblo around. It was home to 85-100 people, and several thousand more lived within a day's walk. And it was built in one of the lowest, warmest, and driest places on the Colorado Plateau.

For a time, in the 1100s, this landscape was densely populated.
The eruption of nearby Sunset Crater Volcano a century earlier probably played a part. Families that lost their homes to ash and lava had to move. They discovered that the cinders blanketing lands to the north could hold moisture needed for crops.

As the new agricultural community spread, small scattered homes were replaced by a few large pueblos, each surrounded by many smaller pueblos and pithouses. Trade networks expanded, bringing exotic items like turquoise, shell jewelry, copper bells, and parrots. Wupatki flourished as a meeting place of different cultures.

Sunset Crater Volcano National Monument

Mailing Address:
6400 U.S. 89
Flagstaff, AZ 86004

Phone: 928-526-0502
Website: www.nps.gov/sucr/index.htm

Roughly 900 years ago, the eruption of this volcano reshaped the surrounding landscape, forever changing the lives of people, plants and animals. Hike the trail through the lava flow and cinders and you'll likely discover colorful, ruggedly dramatic geological features coexisting with twisted Ponderosa Pines and an amazing array of wildlife.

Sunset Crater is a cinder cone located north of Flagstaff in U.S. State of Arizona. The crater is within the Sunset Crater Volcano National Monument. Sunset Crater is the youngest in a string of volcanoes that s related to the nearby San Francisco Peaks.

Sunset Crater Volcano was born in a series of eruptions sometime between 1040 and 1100 CE. Powerful explosions profoundly affected the lives of local people and forever changed the landscape and ecology of the area.

People had been living here for several hundred years, at least, before the volcano erupted. Although we don't know what they called themselves, archeologists consider them representatives of the Sinagua culture. They were farmers, living in scattered groups adjacent to their corn fields. Their homes were pithouses, dug partially into the ground.

Nine hundred years later, Sunset Crater is still the youngest volcano on the Colorado Plateau. The volcano's red rim and the dark lava flows seem to have cooled and hardened to a jagged surface only yesterday. As plants return, so do the animals that use them for food and shelter. And so, do human visitors, intrigued by this opportunity to see natures response to a volcanic eruption.

Montezuma's Castle National Monument

Mailing Address:
P. O. Box 219
Camp Verde, AZ 86322

Phone: 928-567-3322 Ext - #221
Website: www.nps.gov/moca/index.htm

Montezuma Castle National Monument protects a set of well-preserved Ancestral Puebloan cliff dwellings near the town of Camp Verde, Arizona. The dwellings were built and used by the Sinagua people, a pre-Columbian culture closely related to the Hohokam and other indigenous peoples of the southwestern United States, between approximately 1100 and 1425 AD.

Nestled into a towering limestone cliff, the main structure comprises five stories and twenty rooms, and was built over the course of three centuries, that tells a story of ingenuity, tenacity, ingenuity, survival and ultimately, prosperity in an unforgiving desert landscape.

For mysterious and unknown reasons, the Sinagua abandoned its habitat in the 1400's. Maybe they had over extended agricultural pressure on the land. Perhaps there was an unbearable prolonged drought, or most could have been eliminated through conflict with ancient Yavapai Indians. Most Sinaguans likely they were absorbed into other Tribes to the north. The Hopi Indians of today believe they are the descendants of the Sinagua.

Early settlers to the area assumed that the imposing structure was connected to the Aztec emperor Montezuma, but this "castle" was abandoned almost a century before Montezuma was born.

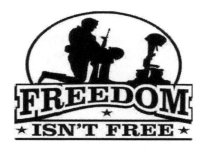

Walnut Canyon National Monument

Mailing Address:
6400 U.S. 89
Flagstaff, AZ 86004

Phone: 928-526-3367
Website: www.nps.gov/waca/index.htm

Walnut Canyon National Monument is located about 10 miles southeast of downtown Flagstaff, Arizona, near Interstate 40. The canyon rimelevation is 6,690 feet; the canyon's floor is 350 feet lower. A 0.9-mile-long loop trail descends 185 feet into the canyon passing 25 cliff dwelling rooms constructed by the Sinagua, a pre-Columbian cultural group that lived in Walnut Canyon from about 1100 to 1250 CE. Other contemporary habitations of the Sinagua people are preserved in the nearby Tuzigoot and Montezuma Castle National Monuments.

Come gaze across curved canyon walls! Among the remarkable geological formations of the canyon itself, the former homes of ancient inhabitants are easily evident. Along the trails, you can imagine life within Walnut Canyon, while visiting actual pueblos and walking in the steps of those who came before.

Hike down into Walnut Canyon and walk in the footsteps of the people that lived here over 900 years ago. Under limestone overhangs, the Sinagua built their homes. These single-story structures, cliff dwellings, were occupied from about 1100 to 1250 CE. The people that lived here moved on to become the modern pueblo people of today. Walnut Canyon is one of their ancestral homes. Walnut Canyon also hosts a vibrant natural environment.

Come out and see millions of years of history unraveled in the geology of the rocks. Listen to the canyon wren and enjoy the turkey vultures soaring above. And if you look closely, you may even see an elk or a javelina. Different life zones overlap here, mixing species that usually live far apart. In this canyon, desert cacti grow alongside mountain firs.

Stand at the Walnut Canyon observation point and gaze across these canyon walls and imagine what life was like for the ancient Sinagua Indians that that once lived in the cliff dwellings at Walnut Canyon. For reasons that are a mystery, they left Walnut Canyon about 800 years ago.

Take a hike along Rim or Island Trails and enter some of cliff dwellings and see many others nestled into the alcoves of the canyon walls.

Tuzigoot National Monument

Mailing Address:
P.O. Box 219
Camp Verde, AZ 86322

Phone: 928-634-5564
Website: www.nps.gov/tuzi/index.htm

The name 'Tuzigoot' is an Apache word meaning "crooked water". Tuzigoot National Monument preserves a 2- to 3-story pueblo ruin on the summit of a limestone and sandstone ridge just east of Clarkdale, Arizona, 120 feet above the Verde River floodplain. The Tuzigoot Site is an elongated complex of stone masonry rooms that were built along the spine of a natural outcrop in the Verde Valley. The central rooms stand higher than the others and they appear to have served public functions. The pueblo has 110 rooms.

Construction of Tuzigoot spanned over 300 years, from about 1100 to 1400 AD. The earliest construction consisted of a small number of rooms near the top of the hill, with new rooms added in an ad-hoc fashion as the population increased.

At its peak, probably in the late 1300's, the pueblo was 500 feet long and 100 feet wide, and contained 86 ground floor rooms and 15 second story rooms and 9 third story rooms, and probably housed as many as 230 people.

The Sinagua, who were the pueblo's occupants, were agriculturalists with trade connections that spanned hundreds of miles. The people left the area around 1400 for reasons unknown. The site is currently comprised of 42 acres.

Discounts Offered by Stores, Services and Online Sites

"The battle, sir, is not the strong alone; it is to the vigilant, the active, and the brave." - Patrick Henry

Though members of the US Military can never be paid/thanked enough for their service to our country, there are many stores and restaurants that attempt to give their daily "thanks" by offering special discounts to active, reserve and retired members of the military.

Here is a list of stores and services doing their part to make life easier by offering discounts to active, reserve, and retired members of the U.S. Military and their immediate family members. There are two important pieces of information for this list. First, some stores offer discounts only at the owner's discretion and other discounts vary by state. Second, many stores that give a military discount don't advertise it. It is always worth asking a store whether they have a discount or not and to have your military ID card on you.

24 Hour Fitness Membership - Active duty military members pay no initiation fee and only pay first and last months' dues in order to open a membership with 24-hour fitness.

99 Restaurants - 10% discount with military ID for active and retired veterans.

1st in Flowers - Send your love home and say it with flowers. With the special 15% military discount, you can show your loved ones that you care at a fraction of the regular price.

A&W - Discount varies, simply ask and have a valid military ID card with you

Abercrombie & Fitch - 10 to 15 % off, at manager's discretion

Acapulco - 20 % off military personnel in uniform or with valid ID card

Acura - $750 military discount

Advance Auto Parts - 10% off regularly price items for in-store purchases to customers who serve or have served our country's Armed Forces. Must show a valid military ID.

63

ACE Rent A Car Military Discount - Get 15% off on car rentals at select ACE Rent A Car locations

AC Lens - Active Duty military members and veterans receive 10% off contact lenses purchased through AC Lens. The promo code MILITARY must be entered during checkout in order to receive the discount.

ACU Army - 5% discount for all. Use discount code "ARMYACU10". Military Clothing, Combat Boots, ACU Uniforms, ACU Coats, ACU Trousers, ACU Patches, TRU Combat Shirts, and Tactical Gear.

Aeropostale - 10% discount with valid military ID card.

Agentsource.com - Up to 40 % off standard real estate closing costs for Active duty men and women moving in the United States or Canada

Alamo Car Rental - Members of the military and their families receive discounted rates through Alamo Car Rental. Those traveling on military orders also receive a Collision Damage Waiver and no additional driver fees.

Alfred Angelo Bridal Gown Discount for Military Brides - Save 15% on a bridal gown at any Alfred Angelo Bridal Boutique. Many locations throughout the U.S.

Aloft Hotels - You can receive a government rate when you book online. You are required to show military ID when you check-in.

American Family Insurance - Active duty service members and veterans who have faced a lapse in insurance due to a deployment are eligible to apply for coverage through American Family Insurance as continuous customers or as having prior insurance. This distinction allows military members to qualify for lower premiums.

AmericInn - Get discounted hotel rates in any of 220 branches nationwide. Simply present a valid US military ID upon check-in.

American Airlines, American Eagle, and American Connections - May offer Military Discount Fares in some markets. These offers include discounted airfares, reduced minimum stay requirements, and preferred boarding privileges. American Airlines currently offers several special discounts that are available exclusively for active duty members of the U.S. Military. These offers include discounted airfares, relaxed advance purchase requirements, and preferred boarding privileges. In addition, the discounted military fares may be purchased up to a week after reservations are made – versus 24 hours for most non-military discount fares – making it easier for military personnel and their families to make travel arrangements. For more information, please call American Airlines Reservations at 1-800-433-7300.

American Airlines Cargo - Ship your pets for 50% less than the regular published rates. Active members of the US Armed Forces as well as their dependents may avail of this discount, which applies to animal shipping for personal use only.

American Car Craft - Enter promo code 'HERO-20' to receive 20% off custom stainless-steel auto accessories, online only at www.americancarcraft.com

American Eagle Outfitters - Offers a 10 % discount when you show your valid military ID.

Amtrak - 10 % off with membership in Veterans Advantage Program

AMC Theaters - After 4 p.m. show your military ID card and get a much-deserved discount on movie tickets.

AmunWave Tactical Optics - 10% off total purchase for all Active Duty Service Members. AmunWave Tactical Optics LLC is a distributor of Numa Sunglasses. AmunWave specializes in tactical, ballistic and sport eyewear.

Anchor Blue - 10 % military discount.

Anheuser – Busch Amusement Parks - Discount varies, simply ask and have a valid military ID card with you

Anna's Linens - 10 % off any purchase with a valid military ID. In-store only. Get 10% off on purchased items by calling 1-866-266-2728 before ordering online.

Anheuser Busch - The Here's to the Heroes Program offers a complimentary single-day admission to SeaWorld, Sesame Place or Busch Gardens for military members and up to three dependents.

Antique Jewelry Mall - With a valid military ID or military e-mail address, military members receive 5% off all jewelry purchases. You must place your order by phone, Skype or e-mail to receive the discount.

Apple Store - Discount varies per location. You need to sign up at www.apple.com/r/store/government. The Apple Federal Government and Military Employee Purchase programs is available to Military personnel, National Guard and Reserve, and their families, along with employees of the federal government. You can get a military discount on iPhones, iPads, iPods and Macs through Apple's Military/Government Purchase Program.

Arby's - Discount varies per location, simply ask and have a valid military ID card with you

Applebee's - Applebee's offers 10% discounts and free meals on Veterans Day at participating locations. Must present valid military ID.

Arizona Art Alliance - Offers free art classes for veterans of all ages. Contact John Fontana (Veterans Programs Manager), at john.fontana@aartalliance.com or at 602-369-2854.

Armed Forces Eyewear - Discounts are offered on eyeglasses, sunglasses and contact lenses for active duty and retired military members and their families.

Armed Forces Vacation Club - The Armed Forces Vacation Club allows active duty and retired military members to book 7-night accommodations for only $349 a week to help them reconnect with family members after a deployment or long stint in the military.

A Story Before Bed - Military members facing deployment are eligible to receive a free recordable storybook.

Ashford University - Discounted tuition at $250 per credit, books are covered for all required courses, waived application fee, waived technology fee and more! Benefits apply to all Active duty, National Guard, Reservists, and spouses, dependents eligible for survivor benefits, plus civilian DOD employees and separated veterans and retirees still using their GI Bill

ASMBA - Armed Services Mutual Benefits Association – Membership in the non-profit association is free, and, when you join, you will get $3,000 of free AD&D coverage

AT&T - Offers 15% monthly service charge discount available to active and retired military personnel, 2-year contract required. Handset pricing: Business 2-year equipment price or best retail offer. Standard IRU validation requirements; must show valid government ID at retail point of sale or validate online with a recognized government email domain (gov. mil et al.) via our online eCommerce site. Military Fan Code: Army – 2421660; Navy – 2421954; Air Force – 2421652; Marines – 2421958; Coast Guard – 2422480.

Audi of America - Get special offers and benefits exclusively available to overseas US military personnel via Audi's Military Sales Program. Visit their website for more info.

Audio Geeks - Active duty, Veterans, Retirees, Reservists and Dependents receive a 15% discount. Use promo code: USMIL15 at check-out.

Auto Accessories Garage - Offers 5 to 20% off to veterans and active duty military plus their families.

Auto Zone - Discount varies per store, simply ask and have a valid military ID card with you

Avis Car Rental - Get special offers and benefits exclusively available to overseas US military personnel via Audi's Military Sales Program. Visit their website for more info.

Award Tech Remote PC Specialists - 10% discount on computer support services for Active Duty, Veterans, Retirees and Reservists. Acceptable ID includes a .mil email address or honor system. No military discount website information available, submitted by business to Military Benefits.

Azamara Cruises – Discounts vary. Call 1-800-338-4962 for details

Baby Direct Military Discount Program - Military staff and family are eligible to receive a 10% discount. Online orders are accepted but you must send a copy of your military ID or other proof of valid service. Must sign up for the program.

Backyard Burgers - Discount varies, simply ask and have a valid military ID card with you

Banana Republic - Offers a flat 10% off for veterans every day.

Bally's Las Vegas - 10% simply ask and have a valid military ID card with you.

Barnes and Noble - 6 % off regular price plus free shipping. Check out www.bn.com/militarycity for more details

Barnhill's - Discount varies, simply ask and have a valid military ID card with you

Baseball Hall of Fame - Free admission year-round for active duty and retired military.

BaseNetOps.Net - Nothing is as comforting as a conversation with loved ones while overseas. Forget about expensive overseas calls and save up to 80% on your phone bill with these affordable military phone cards you can use when calling to and from locations as far as Iraq or Afghanistan.

Bass Pro Shops - For one week, beginning the 15th of every month, active duty and retired military members receive a 10% discount. Some items, such as reels and firearms, are not included.

Bath and Body Works - Discount varies, simply ask and have a valid military ID card with you

Beaches by Sandals - U.S and Canada Military members and their families save an extra 10% at Beaches resorts.

Bed and Breakfast Inns - On November 10th some Arizona Bed and Breakfast Inns are offering a free night's stay to veterans. Others offer discounted rates all year-round. Must call to find out more information. (There is a section later in this book on Bed and Breakfast Inns).

Bed, Bath, and Beyond - Offers a 10% discount for veterans and their families. Discount does vary from store to store, so just ask and have your military ID.

Bennigan's - Active duty and veterans get 10% off their total check at Bennigan's.

Ben & Jerry's - Ask about it next time you order a scoop of ice cream. Discount varies by location, but it is typically 15%.

Berklee School of Music - Get a world-class musical education at a lower price and a more flexible schedule. Active duty and veteran military personnel get a 20% tuition fee discount, on top of available tuition assistance program for military students or GI Bill benefits for veterans. For more details, send an email to registrar@berkleemusic.com or call 1-866-BERKLEE.

Best Bully Sticks - Get discounts on cat and dog supplies by sending an email to bbinfo@bestbullysticks.com from your US military email address. You will be sent a promo code that you can use to get discounted rates.

Best Buy - Discounts vary, simply ask and have a valid military ID card with you.

Best Inns and Suites - Discount varies. Must present a valid military ID card at check-in

Best Western - Rates within allowable per diem, must present a valid military ID card at check-in. Provides hotel rates based on the U.S. government per diem. Available to military personnel or civilian and government employees on official business or leisure.

Big 10 Tires - Discount varies, simply ask and have a valid military ID card with you.

Birdies for the Brave - Complimentary admission for Active, Reserves and military Retirees and dependents at select PGA Tour, Champions Tour, and Web.com Tour Events. Many tournaments also offer discounted admission or complimentary admission for non-retired military veterans. For more information, go to www.birdiesforthebrave.com

Blockbuster - Discount varies, simply ask and have a valid military ID card with you

Blue Star Museums - Members of the Blue Star Museum program offer free admission to military members and their families from Memorial Day to Labor Day. Visitors must present a military ID for free admission.

Bob Evan's - 10% discount with your veterans' ID card.

Boscov's - 15 % off in-store purchases with a valid military ID card everyday

Boston Bill Sunglasses - 10 % off with valid military ID card

Boston Market - Veterans Advantage members to receive 20 % discount at all Boston Market® locations.

Brake Masters - 10% discount at most locations

Brides Across America Military Bride Wedding Gown Giveaway - Bridal retailers and wedding dress designers work with this organization to provide free wedding dresses to military brides. Special wedding dress events are held throughout the year where they giveaway wedding dresses. Check out their site for a listing of the next free wedding dress event in a city near you.

Buckle - The Buckle Military Discount requires online verification. Once verified, you'll get 10% off all purchases.

Budget Car Rental - With the offer code BCD U088801, military members receive discounted rates when booking a rental car online. Discount varies up to 25% off time and mileage. This is in-store only and requires you to show a military ID to redeem.

Budget Truck Rental - Discount varies, simply ask and have a valid military ID card with you.

BuildASign.com - When nothing says it better than a grand gesture, get a free banner or jumbo card to show some big love for troops at home and overseas.

Busch Gardens - (Tampa, FL) Under "Waves of Honor" program, all active duty military are entitled to a free 1-day admission. Also, good for up to 3 family members.

Buffalo Wild Wings - Many Buffalo Wild Wings offer a 10% discount, check with the store first. Typically, you must present a valid military ID.

Burger King - Some participating locations offer 10% discounts, check with the store first. Typically, you must present a valid military ID.

Cabela's - Offers a 5% military discount except on firearms.

Caesar's Atlantic City - 10% must show a valid military ID.

California Coast University - Active duty service members and veterans, as well as their spouses and children, may enjoy 10% discounts on tuition fees. Choose from any of the flexible online degrees in the fields of Business Administration, Marketing, Management, Human Resource Management, Criminal Justice, Education, Psychology or Health Care Administration.

California Southern University - Spouses and children of active-duty and retired military service members can get 10% off on tuition fees for online degree programs in business, psychology and law.

Camp Jellystone - Get up to 20% off campsites, cabins, and more across the country. Must show a valid military ID.

CAM Solar - Reduce your carbon footprint, save energy and save on your electric bill by having solar panels installed in your home. Military discounts are available. Contact 210-227-3456 for details.

Captain D's - Discount varies, simply ask and have a valid military ID card with you

Carl's Jr - Discount varies, simply ask and have a valid military ID card with you

Carnival Cruises - All cruise lines owned by Carnival (Carnival, Princess, Cunard, P & O, etc.) offer free on-board credit for military service, current or past. Just fax them a copy of your discharge papers and you get credit
on any cruise you take with them.

Central Michigan University - National Guard and reserve; active duty military spouses and dependent children; military retirees; honorably discharged veterans; and Department of Defense (DoD) employees may be eligible for discounted tuition fees for undergraduate or graduate degree programs. This applies to both on-campus and online courses.

Century 21 - FREE Century 21 AON Home Protection Plan when you buy or sell a home through Molly Kucharski ONLY. Paid for at settlement. Value $399.00. Call 1-800-952-2516

Champs Sports - Discount varies, simply ask and have a valid military ID card with you

Chase - Free safety deposit box and no fee checking

Chevy Fresh Mex - Military members who visit Chevy's in uniform and present a valid military ID receive 20% off. Discount varies by location.

Chick-Fil-A - Many Chick-fil-A locations offer 10% discounts, always check with the store first. Typically, you must present a valid military ID.

Choice Hotels - Along with discounted rates at over 2,700 hotels, military members and veterans have the option to join the Choice Privileges program as Elite Gold members. This membership entitles them to exclusive benefits and rewards points.

Chipotle - Discount varies and have a valid military ID card with you

Christopher & Banks - 10 % off with valid military ID card

Chrysler - Honoring those who served with $500 bonus cash. This special offer is for those who've risked their lives defending the U.S. If you're active, active reserve, retired military, retired military reserve or are an honorably discharged veteran within twelve months of discharge date, you're eligible for up to $500 in military bonus cash under the Military Incentive Program. Get exclusive rebates and affordable financing deals on Chrysler, Dodge, Jeep and Ram vehicles through the Chrysler Military Program. This offer is available to overseas military personnel.

Ci-Ci's Pizza - Discount varies, dependent on location, must present valid military ID card.

Cinnabon - 15 % off at participating locations with a valid military ID card

Cinemark Movie Theaters - Active military members may get discounted rates upon presenting valid active duty military ID at the ticket booth of selected theaters nationwide. Different terms may apply at each location.

Clipper Vacations Pacific Northwest Travel - Using the promo code HERO while booking online, members of the military and one guest receive discounts on vacation packages in the Pacific Northwest.

Coldstone Creamery - Discount varies and have a valid military ID card with you

CoinsAndPins.com - 10 % military discount on custom made products as long as the custom items are more than 60 % military related

Coleman - 15 % off with Veterans Advantage membership

Continental Airlines - U.S. Active Duty Military, Veterans, National Guard and Reserve, plus their families can get up to 5% discount on airline tickets booked online (continental.com) for Continental and United Airlines-operated flights, with a Veterans Advantage card.

Copeland's Sports - Discount varies, simply ask and have a valid military ID card with you

Costco Wholesale - Join Costco as a new member and receive over $50 in savings for all Members of the Armed Forces, Veterans and their families.

Cotton Patch - Some locations offer a military discount for active duty personnel, Reservists, and retirees. As for Veterans, you will need to ask and present your military ID.

Cracker Barrel - 10 to 15 % off, at manager's discretion

Cube Smart - Active duty military members receive 20% off storage services for the duration of their military service. A copy of deployment orders and a military ID are required.

Culver's Family Restaurant - They generally offer a 10% discount when you show your military ID.

Dairy Queen - Most Dairy Queen locations offer military discounts. The amount varies by location, but may be as high as 50% off for members who show up in uniform.

Day's Inn - Rates within allowable per diem depending on location. Discounts may vary and depend on availability. Must present military ID card

Defense Mobile - Military, veterans and their families get a free SIM card, unlimited talk and text and 1GB of data for b$35/month

Dell - Dell's Military Rewards program offers discounts on laptops that are part of Dell's premier selection. All computers are equipped with webcams to keep military members connected to their families.

Del Taco - 50 % off at participating locations with a valid military ID card

Delta Vacations - Plan your next big trip anywhere in the world and save $50 to $200 on your vacation package of choice. All you need is a valid US military email address to get the discount, along with other perks such as discounted flights and bonus mileage points.

Denny's - Discount varies, simply ask and have a valid military ID card with you

Dick's Sporting Goods - Offers a 10% discount when you show a valid military ID.

Discovery Channel Store - Discount varies, simply ask and have a valid military ID card with you

Discover Credit Card - Discover card holders earn 2% cash back on all purchases at U.S. Military Bases. Instead of receiving a rewards check, members have the option of donating their rewards to Operation Homefront to help other military families.

Disney Parks - Spend a magical day with your loved ones with discounted rates on rooms and admission tickets in Walt Disney World Resort or Disneyland Resort. Active military and spouses, retired military, National Guard and Reservists and their families are eligible for this discount.

Disney Cruise Lines - In honor of the brave men and women who serve this country, Disney Cruise Line is proud to offer special military rates on select Disney cruises through December 2013.

Disney Resorts - Discount varies, simply ask and have a valid military ID card with you

Disneyland - Military discounts are available only for the tickets purchased at installation MWR's. Prices vary per date and length of visit

Dollar.com - Veterans, active duty military, National Guard and Reserve and their families may get amazing discounts in car rentals, as well as fee waivers and other membership rewards. This applies to Veterans Advantage card holders.

Dollywood - Offers a 30% discount on one-day admission tickets for U.S. active duty or retired military, disabled veterans, and military reservists, spouses and dependents when valid military ID's are presented.

Door to Door Storage - Military members receive up to 50% off regular rates from Door to Door storage to help military members who are relocating or transitioning back into civilian life

Dream Stone - By entering the code USTROOPS in the discount box when checking out, military members receive discounts on engagement rings.

Dress Barn - Discount and participation will vary by location. Simply ask and have a valid military ID card with you

DSW Shoe Warehouse - 10% off with a valid military ID.

Dunkin' Donuts - Military members who join Veterans Advantage receive special discounts and promotions on the company's coffee. Dunkin' Donuts also donates coffee to troops serving overseas.

Eastbay - 20 % off on-line and by phone with Veterans Advantage membership

EarthFare - All active duty and reserve military members and their families receive 10% off.

Eddie Bauer - Offers a 10% discount for active and retired military personnel. Must show a valid military ID.

Eders.com - Active duty, retired or honorably discharged members of the US Military get FREE membership to the Professional Bow Hunter Buyer's Club. Members are entitled to anywhere from about 5% to 45% when purchasing archery and bow hunting equipment from eders.com or bowhuntingoutlet.com. Call 516-656-0808 for more details.

Ellis University - A side from tuition fee assistance for online degrees for US military members and their families, Ellis Online University also offers educational counseling, in order to maximize students' learning experience and career opportunities.

Empire Beauty School - Free haircuts

Express Clothing Store - 10 % off on top of other coupons as well with a valid military ID card

Extreme Outfitters - 10 to 20 % off on military gear, on-line and in-store

Eyewear - Discount varies. Get the discount on-line at www.afeyewear.com This site offers military discounts for a wide range of eyeglass companies

Facets Collection - 10 % off jewelry and 5 % off all engagement rings and loose diamonds

Fathead - 20 % off all Fathead products, every day. Open to United States Active duty and Retired service members, veterans and members of their immediate families

Famous Footwear - Offers a 10% discount to all members of the U.S. Armed Forces and their families. In-store ONLY and may not be combined with any other coupons. It is valid with Rewards certificates and BOGO ½ off. To get the discount, a current, valid government issued military ID card must be presented at time of purchase.

Famous Dave's BBQ - All active duty & retired military can get a 10% discount. Just ask for it.

Fandango - The availability of discounted military tickets is controlled by each individual theater, not by Fandango. To see if any discounts are being offered for your theater for purchases made via Fandango, click on a red show time to begin the purchase process. All available ticket categories will be displayed on the subsequent page. Look for ticket categories labeled "military discount" or similarly named categories which would indicate a specially priced ticket. Also, not all theaters that offer military discounts make them available through Fandango.

Finish Line - 20 % military discount off select items at special locations

FlowerShop.com - This online florist offers specially designed military care packages that may be shipped to APO/FPO addresses as well.

Foot Action - 20 % off with a valid military ID card

Foot Locker - 20 % off with a valid military ID card

Ford - Ford Motor Company is honored to reward commitment to our country through the exclusive Military Appreciation Program. This offer provides the opportunity to receive a special offer good toward the purchase or lease of any eligible new Ford car, truck, or SUV through F-550 (excluding Mustang Shelby GT, Shelby GT 500, Harley and Hybrid Vehicles. Other restrictions may apply).

Ford Mobility Motoring - At Ford we have a lend commitment to making it easier for persons with disabilities (and those who care for them) to purchase and adopt vehicles to fit their individual wants and needs. Go to their website: www.fordmobilitymotoring.com

Forever 21 - 10 % off with a valid military ID card

Frame of Choice - 35% off prescription eyewear and accessories. Call 1-800-227-6342 to verify and receive your discount code.

Fred Meyer Jewelers - 10% off. Some restrictions may apply

Freedom Furniture and Electronics - Get $100 off on computers, HDTV's, dining sets, living room sets, and Sealy Posturepedic mattresses. Visit www.shopfreedom.com or call 888-480-4015 for orders or inquiries.

Friendly's Ice Cream Stores - Discount varies, simply ask and have a valid military ID card with you

FromYouFlowers.com - 20 % discount when you order by phone at 1-800-838-8853

Fuddruckers - Discounts vary by location, but range from 10-15% off for those who present a military ID.

Gander Mountain - 5 % off with a valid military ID card

Gap - 10 % off military discount 1st of every month (may vary by location; in-store ONLY)

General Motors - Active Duty members, reserves and retirees, including their spouses, of the U.S. Air Force, Army, Navy, Marines, National Guard and Coast Guard can save hundreds or even thousands of dollars when purchasing eligible Chevrolet, Buick or GMC vehicles through the GM Military Discount Program. There are also regional and dealership incentives available.

Geico - Pay 15% less than regular insurance premiums if you are an active duty or retired member of the military, or a member of the National Guard or Reserves.

Gift Express - 20% discount on fine personalized gifts, personalized stationery gifts & gifts for business. Use code USA for 20% savings with a minimum purchase of $39.95. Shipping to APO addresses as well.

GlassesUSA.com - Save up to 15% on eyewear ordered online. Use promo code MilSpouse15.

GNC - Discount varies, simply ask and have a valid military ID card with you

Go Baby Go - 10% military discount. Present proof of a valid Military, Police or Fire ID and receive 10% off your initial order and a coupon code of 10% for all future orders. Conditions apply, see site or details.

Goettl Air Conditioning - Offers a 5% discount on all services for active duty military and veterans.

Good Sam RV Club - Free membership

Gold's Gym - Gold's Gym offers free enrollment for members of the military. In most locations members also receive $10 off their monthly dues.

Golden Corral - Discount varies, simply ask and have a valid military ID card with you

Goodwill - Stores hold Military Discount Days throughout the year where military members receive 10% off. The exact day varies by location.

Goody's - Discount varies, simply ask and have a valid military ID card with you.

Great Wolf Lodge & Indoor Water Park - Great Wolf Lodge, with suites and an indoor water park offers a 10% discount for military members, retired military and their families. Book online using the offer code HEROES. It is limited to two suites per military ID or badge and based upon availability. A valid ID or badge is required at check in. Police, Fire and EMS workers can also take advantage of this discount.

Greyhound - Get a 10% discount on fares for you and your family if you are either active duty or retired US military personnel. Other terms may apply.

Group Health Eye Care - Military members and veterans receive 20% off prescription eyeglasses and contact lenses.

GuideToMilitaryTravel.com - Military families can get great discounts on selected travel destinations within the country. Be ready to provide valid identification and/or documents.

Haber Vision - Protect your eyes from the sun's harmful rays and prevent wrinkles caused by squinting too much in the sunlight with Haber Vision sunglasses. Military personnel can get a pair for half the regular retail price.

Hanes Outlet Store - 10 % off with a valid military ID card

Hardees - 10% discount. Just show your valid military ID.

Hard Rock Café - All Hard Rock Café locations offer a year-round 15% discount for military members who present a valid military ID. That discount is increased to 20% during select months.

Harley-Davidson - Military personnel serving outside the US can take advantage of the Harley-Davidson Military Sales Program to get discounts on a large selection of Harleys. With a no down payment program along with reduced rates and flexible term options designed specifically for active duty military personnel.

Harrah's - 10% simply ask and have a valid military ID card with you.

Helzberg Diamonds - 10% discount to all active military when placing an order over the phone at 1-800-HELZBERG (435-9237); M-F 8am-5pm CST. Most Helzberg locations honor the military discount as well but call ahead to confirm. Proof of ID required before processing the discount.

Hertz Rental Cars - Members of the military receive discounted rates and unlimited mileage through Hertz Rental Cars. Free upgrades are also offered if space is available.

Hewlett Packard - HP offers a military discount program with up to 10% off computers and other special promotions. Military members must sign-up for the program to access the discounts. Log on to website and click on New User Registration: Enter first and last name, username, password and email address. Use company code: 2727. discounts vary. On-line ONLY.

HickoryFarms.com - 10 % military discount. Enter 892848 in code box on-line order form. Send gifts to APO and FPO addresses – shipping is free.

Hi-Health Innovations - Hearing aid discount for veterans – starting at $649 each

Hilton Hotels - Offers a 10% discount on leisure stays for active duty and retired military and their families at participating hotels and resorts.

Home Depot - A year-round 10% discount up to a maximum $500 at all U.S. locations to active duty personnel, reservists, retired or disabled veterans and their immediate families. Must present a valid military ID. A 10% discount is also offered to all other military veterans on Memorial Day, Fourth of July, Labor Day and Veterans

Honda - The Military Appreciation Offer can be used toward the purchase or lease of any new Honda automobile using a valid Honda APR, Honda Leadership Lease®, or Honda Leadership Purchase Plan® program through HFS (excludes Zero Due at Signing established by HFS, and the vehicle must be eligible for new-vehicle rates.

Hooters - Discounts varies by locations but most locations will give a flat 15% off discount to active duty personnel and retired military personnel. Other times, the discount is only available on certain nights.

Howard Johnson's – Discount of about 10 %. Rate depends on availability. Must present military I.D. upon check in.

Hot Topic - Get 10-20% off on purchases by calling 1-800-892.8674 for US customers or 1-626-709-1189 for international customers.

Hypnosis.org - Interested in a career in hypnosis? Apply for a hypnosis certification course and get a 20% discount if you are active duty or veteran military personnel. Call 714-258-8380 or 800-965-3390 to register.

Hyundai - Active duty, veteran or retired members of the US military may get a $500 price slash on any new Hyundai vehicle. Availability is subject to terms, valid until January 4, 2012 to April 2, 2012. Ask your local dealership for more information.

IAVA - IAVA, Iraq and Afghanistan veterans of America, is a veteran's organization that looks to help take care of the newest generation of American veterans. They are also working with companies, such as JC Penny to provide up to $200 in vouchers to certain retail stores

IHOP - 20 % off military ID, at owner's discretion

IMAX - $1.00 off movie tickets with military ID card

Indian Motorcycles - Offers a discount of $1000 off certain motorcycles. Just ask and have a valid military ID.

Infiniti - Receive exclusive new vehicle pricing with the Vehicle Purchase Program. Special pricing varies by month. Must be active duty or Reserves and their dependents (spouse/domestic partner). U.S. Military includes: Army, Navy, Air Force, Marines, Coast Guard and National Guard.

Inkshouse.com - 20 % off $50 or more purchase. Use code Mil20

Java Café - Discount varies, simply ask and have a valid military ID card with you

Jeep - $500 off for Active military, reserves and retired reserves or Active after 20 years of service. Requires a military ID card

Jelly Bean Quilts - 15% discount on all quilts for Active Duty, Veterans, Retirees and Dependents. Memory quilts are made out of baby clothing, t-shirt quilts, and memorial clothing quilts. Email for discount details: contact@jellybeanquilts.com. Discount is based on the honor system. No military discount website information available, submitted by business to Military Benefits.

Jellystone Parks - Active duty and retired military families who enjoy camping receive discounts at most of Jellystone's campgrounds. Discounts range from 5% to 20% off and vary by location.

Jiffy Lube - Most Jiffy Lube locations offer up to 15% off to military members. Because Jiffy Lube locations are independently owned, some may opt not to participate in the discount program.

JC Penny Portraits – Offers a free sitting, an 8X10 print, and 50% off entire purchase

Jockey - 10 % off with military ID card

Johnny Rockets - Personnel in uniform will receive a 50 % discount

Jones New York Outlet Store - 10 % off with military ID card.

KB Toys - 15 % off during advertised military days

KFC - Discount varies, simply ask and have a valid military ID card with you.

Kid's Foot Locker - 20 % off with military ID card

Kiss the Cook - Register with your military email address and receive a 10 % discount

Knott's Berry Farm - Free entry on Memorial Day weekend and substantial discounts the rest of the year.

Kaplan University - Active-duty military service members, their spouses and veterans may avail of discounted tuition fees at Kaplan University, one of the top military-friendly colleges and universities for three consistent years.

Keystone School - Active duty US military families may get up to 10% off on tuition fees for Keystone School's online high school and middle school programs. Call 1-800-255-4937 to enroll. Discounts are not applicable to online enrollments.

KOA Campgrounds - Most KOA campgrounds offer a military discount between 5% and 15% off the regular price. Check with your specific campground to find out the discount it offers.

Kohl's - Get a 15% discount by presenting a valid US military ID in selected Kohl's branches nationwide.

Lady Foot Locker - Active military, veterans and their families can purchase quality athletic footwear at Lady Foot Locker via stores, phone orders and online orders at 20% off. To avail of a discount, one must also be a Veterans Advantage member.

Lamps.com - Military discount of 15 %. Use code: MILITARY15

Land Rover - $750 off new purchase

Larson Jewelers - Active duty military members receive 5% off the purchase of wedding rings and bands

La Quinta Inns & Suites - While it does not publish its military rates, La Quinta Inns & Suites advertises special rates for members of the military who provide a valid ID. Choose the government rate option when booking online.

LEGOLAND - 10% military discount at the California LEGOLAND location. Military Appreciation Days at the Florida location gets active and retired veterans in the park for free with discounts for family members.

Len's Crafters - 30% military discount

Lerner - 15 % off with military ID card

Leslie Pool Supplies - 10 % off with military ID card

Levi's - 25% off on two women's items

Levi's - 30% off new arrivals for men and kids

Life Lock - 15% off identity theft protection for active, retired & family members

Lincoln Motor Company - Active military personnel and Reservists serving on active duty, Veterans separated within the last 180 days, Retirees, Spouses/Surviving Spouses, or other household members are eligible for a $750 Bonus Cash Offer good toward the purchase or lease of an eligible new or recent model year Lincoln vehicle.

Lonestar Steakhouse & Saloon - All veterans and active duty personnel, police and firefighters get a 15% discount every Monday.

Long John Silver's - Discount varies, simply ask and have a valid military ID card with you

Longhorn Steakhouse - 10 % military discount

Lowe's - Lowe's offers a regular 10% military discount to active duty military members and veterans who present a military ID or Veteran Identification Card. Special discounts are also available on military holidays. The military discount, however, cannot be combined with other coupons they may be offering

Kragen Auto Parts - Discount varies, simply ask and have a valid military ID card with you

Macy's - 10 % off on the first Tuesday of every month. 15 % with a Macy's card

Margaritaville - 10 % off with military ID card

Marriott Hotels - Find out how much you can save in hotel rates under Marriott's Military Per Diem Rate Qualification Guidelines.

Mary Kay Cosmetics - Military personnel and dependents receive 10 % on on-line orders. Reference your military affiliation and status, and ask for additional free gift and bigger discounts by contacting website

Massage Envy Military Discount Program - All active-duty military personnel who join Massage Envy get $60 off a year. Call ahead to ensure the location is participating and rates may vary.

Maurice's - 10 % off with military ID card.

Mazda - Active Military can get $500 Bonus Cash toward the purchase or lease of a new Mazda. Limit two purchases per person, per year. The Military Bonus Cash Program CANNOT be combined with other private offers (excluding Owner Loyalty) but CAN be combined with other public purchase incentives including, but not limited to, customer cash back, lease and APR incentives/offers. Must be a U.S. resident. This offer is for a limited time, see your Mazda dealer for details.

McDonalds - Discount varies, simply ask and have a valid military ID card with you

Meineke - 10 % off parts, in-store ONLY. Simply ask and have a valid military ID card with you. Meineke franchises offer discounts to military members on select services. Discounts and qualified services vary by location

MetalDetector.com - MetalDetector.com proudly offers a coupon code 5JJA for a $5 discount off online purchase of $50 or more. Just enter this code at checkout for an instant discount. This "Discounts to Support the Troops" program applies to all service members with an APO/FPO address. Members of the U.S. Army, Navy, Marines, Coast Guard and Air Force have also been given the option of free shipping.

Microsoft Office 2015 - Save up to 45% off the regular retail price on Microsoft Office Home and Student 2010 - Military Appreciation Edition. This all-in-one Office package includes Word 2010, Excel 2010, Powerpoint 2010 and OneNote 2010. Active Duty Military, National Guard personnel, Reserves, US Civilian Department of Defense employees stationed overseas and Department of State officials serving in Foreign countries, as well as their dependents.

Microsoft 365 - All military personnel save up to 30% off Microsoft 365 which includes Microsoft Word, Excel, Outlook, Powerpoint, Skype, SkyDrive, Access, Publisher and OneNote.

Michael's - Offers a flat 10% off when you show your valid military ID.

Midas - 10 % off with a valid military ID card

MilitaryContacts.net - Up to 30 % off contact lenses and free shipping on orders over $50

Military Clothing Stores - Offers a military discount for sub-totals over $50. Use discount code: MILITARY.

Military Cruise Deals - Double discounts on cruises, www.militarycruisedeals.com

Military Resort Deals - Double discounts on Sandals and Beaches resorts, www.militaryresortdeals.com

MLB Hall of Fame - Discount varies, simply ask and have a valid military ID card with you

Modern Furniture for Home - All US military personnel may get 10% off on furniture. Simply fax a copy of an active military ID card to 323-782 0889 or upload a scanned copy through their website, in order to get a coupon code.

Moissante Bridal - Military members receive 5% off the purchase of an engagement ring.

Motel 6 - All military and retired military personnel and their families are eligible for a 10% discount. When booking online, simply click 'Military Rate' before selecting your room type and the discount will be automatically applied.

Movie Theaters - Discount varies, simply ask and have a valid military ID card with you

Mrs. Field's Cookies - 10 % off with military ID card

My Alarm Center - 2 months of free cellular monitoring for veterans and Active military members

NAPA Auto Parts - Discount varies, simply ask and have a valid military ID card with you.

National Association of Photoshop Professionals - Active US military personnel can now learn the coolest Photoshop tips and tricks for $20 less. Be ready to provide proof of active military status.

National Association of Realtors - 5% + $150 service credit

National Car Rental - Military members receive discount rates on car rentals and no additional driver fees when traveling on official military orders.

National Credit Solutions - 25 % discount, call toll free at 1-866-485-2540 x109, and for a direct line call 972-746-4209

Nautica - 10% off at certain locations

Navy Federal Credit Union - Active duty and retired military personnel may qualify for a ¼ % APR discount on selected loans. Call 1-888-842-6328 or visit your nearest NFCU branch. Offer is not available for online applications.

Nerve.org - With a 5% discount on all procedures for military personnel and their spouses, you may save hundreds of dollars upon presenting a valid US military ID or equivalent proof of military status.

New York and Company - 15% off in-store.

Nickelodeon Hotels - Reduced rates and perks, on-line and in-store, www.nickhotel.com/military, or call 1-877-NICK-111 and ask for the Military Family Package

Nickelodeon Suite Resort - This Orlando resort offers 20% off accommodations and 10% off food and beverages through its military appreciation package.

Nike - Active, retired, reservist US military personnel and their families get 10% off in Nike-owned stores including Nike Stores, NikeFactory Stores, NIKETOWN and Nike Women in the US and Puerto Rico. Present a valid US military ID for verification.

Nissan Military Program - Nissan offers a discount for Active Duty Military, Reserves, Retired, or Veteran (best be within 12 months from discharge or retirement. See website: www.nissanusa.com/military for more information.

Norton Antivirus Software - $32 off annual 5 device protection plan

Norwegian Cruise Lines - The military and their families can receive up to 10% off on select cruises. Includes veterans, active duty military, national guard, or reserves.

Nuvo - $30 off Ritmo Pregnancy Sound System. You can call 1-888-688-6462 or use coupon code: MILITARY (on-line at www.nuvo-group.com. Valid military ID card required for in-store purchase

Oakley - There is a website you register with that offers Oakley's at a discounted price. It doesn't say how much that price is though. Check it out on-line at secure.usstandardissue.com. The program is for active duty military, reserve, federal and local law enforcement, fire, EMS and those holding military retiree credentials. Must have a valid .gov or .mil email address entered during registration confirm your approval. The discount is available through their USS Standard Issue Website.

Old Navy - Keep an eye out and ask about Military Monday's, where active and retired military personnel get a 10 – 15% discount.

Operation Homelink - Provides free refurbished computers to the spouses or parents of junior enlisted (E-1 – E-5) U.S. deployed service members enabling email communications with their loved ones deployed overseas.

Operation Love Reunited - Photographers partner with this organization to provide free photo shoots for military members and their loved ones before or after a deployment. landscaping services for military families.

O'Reilly Auto Parts - Offers an "in-store only" discount of 10 – 15% with a valid military ID.

Outback Steakhouse - In addition to providing a free Bloomin' Onion appetizer to all active duty military who show an ID, Outback supports Operation Homefront and other military programs through proceeds from special restaurant promotions.

Orvis - 10 % discount for Veterans Advantage members.

Overstock.com - Free Club O membership for military personnel with a valid .mil email address or active, retired or reserve military. Membership benefits include 5% reward dollars on every purchase, free shipping every day of the year and extra reward dollars on select products.

Panda Express - 10% military discount for active duty. Just show your military ID.

Operation Homelink - Provides free refurbished computers to the spouses or parents of junior enlisted (E-1 – E-5) U.S. deployed service members enabling email communications with their loved ones deployed overseas.

Pac Sun - Discount varies per location, just bring in a valid military ID card with you

Panera Bread - 10% off when not in uniform; 65% in uniform.

Panchero's Mexican Grill - Discount varies, simply ask and have a valid military ID card with you.

Pancho's Mexican Buffet - Discount varies, simply ask and have a valid military ID card with you

Papa Murphey's - Participating locations will take 50 % off one pizza.

Paradise Limousines - $25 off Limousine service, use coupon code: 1369 for service members.

Park-Ride-Fly-USA - Airport parking discounts to all Veterans, Armed Forces personnel and their families.

Paris Las Vegas - 10% have a valid military ID card with you

Payless Shoe Source - All US military personnel and their immediate family members get 10% off on any purchase (on top of other possible discounts and promos) at Payless Shoe Source branches in the United States and Puerto Rico.

Penske Truck Rentals - Get up to 20% off on military relocation packages with a valid military ID. They will also match any price.

Pep Boys Military Discount - Every Tuesday, Wednesday and Thursday active-duty and retired military customers can receive a 10% discount at local stores. Present a valid military or veteran ID to save.

Pizza Hut - Discount varies, simply ask and have a valid military ID card with you

Planet Hollywood Las Vegas - 10% have a valid military ID card with you.

Play It Again Sports - Discount varies, simply ask and have a valid military ID card with you

PODS - Military members and veterans are eligible for discounted storage rates through PODS.

Portrait Innovations - 10% discount on all portrait packages and specialty portrait products for active duty military families.

ProFlowers - Discounts can vary but typically it is 20% off. Anybody can get this discount by visiting the Pro Flowers Military Discount page. You can also visit their promotions page for additional discounts.

ProFox Racing - Adrenaline junkies can get 10% discounts (plus free shipping within the US!) on regular-priced racing gear and accessories. This offer is available for Active Duty, veteran, reserve, Coast Guard, National Guard, retired and military families.

Popeye's - 10 % off with valid military ID card

Professional Sports Teams - Discount varies, simply ask and have a valid military ID card with you.

Pure Beauty - Discount varies, simply ask and have a valid military ID card with you

Purina Care - Military families receive a 5% discount on pet health insurance through Purina Care. Families with two or more pets receive a 10% discount.

Quizno's - Discount varies, simply ask and have a valid military ID card with you.

Race Depot - 10 % off. Use code: 10MILCITY

Rack Room Shoes - Offers a 10 % discount to active duty military personnel and their families every Tuesday plus on Memorial Day, Independence Day, and Veterans Day. Bring in a valid military ID card.

Radiological Society of North America - Actively deployed members of the US Armed Forces can get a membership for half the regular price. This membership gives them full online access to RSNA Journals, Radiology, Radio Graphics and RSNA News, Education Center, CME, SAMs, and complimentary advanced registration to the RSNA Annual Meeting.

Radio Shack - Offers a flat 10% discount to active and retired military. Must show a valid military ID.

Ralph Lauren Outlet Store - 10 % off with military ID card.

Raising Cane's Chicken - Discount varies, simply ask and have a valid military ID card with you.

Ramada - 15 % to 30 % - Depending on availability. Must present a valid military ID card upon check-in.

Red Robin - Discount varies, simply ask and have a valid military ID card with you.

Red Roof Inn - Active duty and retired military members receive 10% off room rates. When booking online, use the VP+(R) code 604287.

Regent University - Get an online degree with very little to no expense. Active-duty military, reservists, and National Guard personnel may qualify for discounted tuition rates, which may usually be covered by military Tuition Assistance. Veterans and retirees may also qualify for discounted rates.

Regal Cinemas - Offers a military discount but varies by location. Inquire at your local theater.

Ripley's Attractions and Museums - Discount varies, simply ask and have a valid military ID card with you.

Rio Las Vegas - 10% have a valid military ID card with you.

RocketLife - Families of active duty military members may create a free 5×7 photo book to ship to any APO, FPO or MPO address.

Rocky Mountain Chocolate Factory - 10 % military discount.

Rocky Mountain Tracking - 5 % off any tracking device. Use code: USMILITARY. www.rmtracking.com

Royal Caribbean -Take advantage of special cruise rates available for military personnel and their family members. Eligible military members must be in the same stateroom in order for dependents to qualify for discounted rates. Discounts are subject to terms.

Ryan Homes - Ryan Homes gives military members access to the Hero's Welcome Home program which provides $1500 for extra home options or to put toward closing costs.

Saint Joseph's University - Active duty and reserve military personnel and their spouses can get tuition fee discounts on graduate or undergraduate degree programs, along with other GI Bill educational benefits.

Sally Beauty Supply - Get a free Beauty Club membership card ($5 value) when you visit a Sally Beauty Supply store and present a valid US military ID. With the card, you get special member pricing on non-sale items and 15% discounts on future purchases.

Sam's Club - Active duty, retired military and civilian military employees and their spouses receive a $15 gift upon joining or renewing a Sam's Club membership.

Samsonite - 15 % off with military ID.

Samuel's Diamonds - 10 % off with military ID.

Satellite Internet Pro's - $100 instant savings on subscribers who decide to purchase a new Hughes Net system, or a $99 savings + free installation on new subscribers who choose to rent the equipment.

Sandal's Vacations - Military members receive 10% off the purchase of all-inclusive vacation. packages from Sandals. The discount is on top of other promotions the company offers.

San Diego Zoo - Free 1-day admission for those who are active duty military.

Schlotzsky's - 20% discount with a valid military ID.

Scion - If you are a member of the U.S. Military with current active duty status or an inactive Reservist, you may qualify for a $500 rebate towards the purchase or lease of a new Scion when financed or leased through a participating Scion dealer and Toyota Financial Services (TFS). Active duty military members may request a free care package from Scion that includes a deck of cards, free hour of Internet access and other swag.

Scorpyd Crossbows - 10% percent discount to all Active, Honorably Discharged and Retired military personnel. Scorpyd will also offer the discount to all active Law Enforcement Officers and all active Fire Department personnel. To receive the discount, you will have to call Scorpyd directly and be able to present a valid document to prove that you are currently Active, Honorably Discharged or Retired from the military. Law Enforcement and Fire Department Personnel will have to present a Department Letter Head to receive the discount. This discount only applies to direct orders from Scorpyd Crossbows.

Sea World - Members of the military and as many as three direct dependents may enter SeaWorld, Busch Gardens or Sesame Place parks with a single-day complimentary admission. Military personnel must register to receive tickets.

Sears Portrait Studio - Discount varies, simply ask and have a valid military ID card with you

Sesame Park Place - One-day complimentary admission for members of the military and 3 direct dependents.

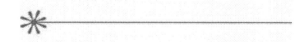

Shades of Green - The Magic Your Way Stars and Stripes Tickets are offered to Shades of Green guests or guests staying at the Walt Disney World Resort. The Magic Your Way Stars and Stripes Tickets includes admission for the specified days to the Magic Kingdom, Epcot, Disney's Hollywood Studios, Disney's Animal Kingdom Theme Park, Blizzard Beach, Typhoon Lagoon, Disney Quest and Wide World of Sports. The current prices for these passes that include Military discounts can be found on www.shadesofgreen.com

Shedd Aquarium in Chicago - Free general admission with military ID. On the Shedd Aquarium page, scroll down to 'Other Discounts' to find out more information.

ShipAnyCar.com - Whether you need your vehicle transported for military relocation or for personal use, you can get a $25 discount on your car transportation fees.

Shoney's - 15 % off for all Service Men and Women in uniform. Military, Fire, Police and EMT's in uniform also qualify. At participating locations

Simone Protective Health - 20 % off their nutritional hydration drink.

Since 1910.com - Ready to pop the big question and put a ring on it? Get 5% off on an engagement ring of your choice (maximum price of $10,000) by simply providing your US military email address.

Sitter City - Members of the military receive free access to Sittercity.com to help them find qualified childcare providers, housekeepers and other service providers in their area.

Six Flags - Check out the website BaseOps.net and collect discounted tickets to all Six Flags properties.

Six Flags Magic Mountain - Six Flags parks offer military appreciation days where military members receive free admission. Days vary by park and season. Additionally, Tickets are available at discounted prices, varies by location, on military bases and installations through the MWR or ITT recreation offices. Quantities are unlimited with a valid military or DoD ID. Discounted tickets are NOT available at the parks.

Sizzler - Discount varies, simply ask and have a valid military ID card with you.

Smith & Wesson - Get as much as $100 worth of rebates on purchased firearms. Active duty U.S. Military, Retired Military with retired Military Status, active National Guard Reservists and Disabled Veterans of all U.S. Military branches including U.S. Coast Guard may all qualified for these rebates upon fulfillment of other documentation requirements.

Sonic - Discount varies, simply ask and have a valid military ID card with you.

SOS Eyewear - Military members receive 25% off sunglasses in the SOS Eyewear Military or US Ranger lines by entering the code MIL25 at checkout.

Southwest Airlines - Varies. It's a dollar amount, not a percentage. Not available on all flights. You will have to call Southwest Airlines and simply ask. up to $250 off Mexico, Caribbean and Costa Rica vacation packages.

Spencer's Gifts - Discount varies, simply ask and have a valid military ID card with you.

Sports Authority - Offers a 10% discount when you show your military ID.

Sport Chalet - 10 % off. Have a valid military ID card with you.

Sport Clips - Active duty military and veterans receive special pricing on haircuts. Prices vary by location. Veterans also receive 10% off Sports Clips franchise fees.

Sportsmemorabilia.com - 10 % off at checkout, use code: mili10 on-line.

Sprint - 10 % to 18 % off. Sprint will also put a 'hold' on your line when you are deployed, if you provide a copy of your orders, so you will still have the same number when you come back and you do not have to pay for the time that you are gone.

Sprint Business - 15 % to 20 % discount. 1-888-788-4727.

Stanton Homes - Through the Stanton Homes for Heroes program, active duty military members and veterans receive 3% off the price of a new home. Some of the companies Stanton homes contracts with offer additional discounts during the homebuilding process.

Starwood Hotels - Active or retired military members and their families may take advantage of the special online rate, or free lessons in its music studio in Arkansas.

Stationary Xpress - 20% discount on personalized stationery, embossed stationery, raised print stationery, raised-print stationery, invitations, announcements, stationery gifts, stationary. Use promo code "USA" for 20% savings with a minimum purchase of $39.95 and shipping to APO addresses.

Studio 09 - Active duty military have the option of booking one room through Starwood Hotels at a discounted rate. In order to receive the rate, a valid military ID must be presented during check-in.

Subway - 10 % off, if not in a military town.

Suncoast - Discount varies, simply ask and have a valid military ID card with you.

Superior Nut - Use coupon code: "Military" for a 10% discount.

Suzuki - $500 off for you and immediate family. Requires a valid military ID.

Sweet Dreams Picture Pillows - Free picture pillow.

Sweet Tomatoes - 10 % off with a valid military ID card. Free shipping to military APO/FPO destinations.

T – Mobile - Switch to T-Mobile and take advantage of America's Largest 4G Network, affordable smartphones, 15% discount on monthly service and waived activation fees. * For additional information or to place a new order, please contact T-Mobile at 1-877-426-2024. Reference promo code #15327TMOFAV. Already using T-Mobile, call 1-877-453-8824 or go to www.tmobile.com/corpdiscount.com to check your eligibility. *(*some restrictions may apply).

Taco Bell - Discount varies, simply ask and have a valid military ID card with you.

Target Portraits - Present your Military ID at time of sitting, along with coupon to receive 50% off portrait collections, one free 8×10 and free sitting fees.

Taylor Made Golf - Offers a 20% discount for Active Duty, Retirees, Veterans, Military Spouses, Military Family Members on these four sites: taylormadegolf.com; adidisgolf.com; ashworthgolf.com; and adamsgolf.com. The discount cannot be combined with other promotional codes and some exclusions may apply.

TBC Retail Group (Tire & Auto Centers) - Spend 10% less on tire and auto services at any of 1,300 Tire Kingdom, NTB-National Tire and Battery, Merchant's Tire and Auto Centers and Big O Tires centers nationwide. Present a valid US military ID to enjoy these discounts.

Texas Roadhouse - Get up to 10% off your bill with your military ID.

The Finish Line - Discount varies, simply ask and have a valid military ID card with you.

The Flamingo Las Vegas - 10% have a valid military ID card with you.

The Heart Rate Watch Company - US military active duty and retired receive 10% off all heart rate monitors, GPS watches and remote charging equipment from brands like Garmin, Sunto, Polar, Times, Goal Zero and more. Shipping is free to APO and a free fitness book is included as well. To get the promo code contact required at heartratewatchcompany.com to or call toll-free at 866-586-7129.

The LINQ Hotel and Casino - 10% military discount.

The Melting Pot - Discount varies, simply ask and have a valid military ID card with you.

The National Parks and Recreational Lands Pass - Available to US military members and their dependents in the Army, Navy, Air Force, Marines, and Coast Guard, as well as most members of the US Reserves and National Guard. Proper military ID is required (CAC Card or DoD Form 1173). Covers entrance to Fish and Wildlife Service and National Park Service sites that charge Entrance Fees, and Standard Amenity Fees at Forest Service, Bureau of Land Management and Bureau of Reclamation sites. In addition, most state and federal parks grant free access on Veteran's Day and other military holidays.

Thrifty.com - Federal government and military personnel can get discounts and other perks on car rentals.

Timberland Outlets - 15 % off, bring in a valid military ID card.

Titus-Will Chevrolet - Get discounts on new and used vehicles as well as easy payment options and instant loan approvals for military personnel.

Tommy Hilfiger - 10 % off, bring in a valid military ID card.

Torrid - Military members receive a 10% discount in Torrid stores or by calling to place an order with a Torrid Personal Shopper.

Tough Mudder Events - $10 rebate off the participant registration price for active and veteran members of the military.

Toyota - Active duty military and reserve members receive a $500 off + $500 for first time buyers. Requires a valid military ID card.

Travelodge - Rate within allowable per diem. Discounts may vary and depend on availability. Must present a valid military ID card.

Trident University - Trident University's Military Discount Program (MDP) covers regular military personnel, drilling and active duty reservists, retired military personnel and members of the National Guard. Military spouses may also qualify for discounts.

Turbo Tax - Active duty military are eligible to file federal tax returns for free through the Intuit Tax Freedom Project

Tutor.com - Free Tutoring for Military Families. Army, Air Force, Navy, Marines and National Guard and Reserve military families can receive free online tutoring. See website for details.

Under Armour Military Discount - Present a valid US military ID at any Under Armour store and get a 10% off on your purchase. Get 10% off everything for Veterans & Service Members at UnderArmour.com! Plus, for a limited time get free shipping.

United Postal Service (USPS) - The Postal Service offers free Mili-Kits that contain all the supplies needed for shipping items to military members overseas.

United Airlines - Offers reduced domestic fares. These fares are for U.S. Military personnel and their eligible family members who are traveling on leave. Military personnel and eligible dependents must have a valid military ID and must use personal credit cards for payment. Authorized federal government credit cards will not be accepted for payment of military leisure fares. For more information, see the website www.united.com

US Airways - Offers special military discount rates to military personnel traveling on an officially excused absence and to discharged personnel within seven days of discharge. Special rates are also applicable for military dependents. Special rates are not available to personnel on temporary duty orders traveling to or from their temporary duty station. For more information about Military Leave Travel, call US Airways at 1-800-428-4322.

USAA - USAA provides discounted auto, home and life insurance to military members and veterans. Since the insurance is only available to those who have served in the military, no additional military discounts are offered.

United Artists Movie Theater - Matinee show prices for all show times. Requires a valid military ID card.

Universal Studios - Offers phenomenal discount options to all members of our Armed Forces all year long! Eligible members include active duty, retirees, DOD personnel, members of the National Guard/Reserves, dependents and all other base personnel. Tickets for these specially priced offers must be purchased in advance and can only be obtained at participating MWR ITT/ITR offices throughout the United States. These special military rates are NOT available at the Universal Studios Hollywood box office. A military or U.S. Government ID is required for purchase.

USA RV Rentals - Active duty members and veterans may rent affordable motor homes from USA RV Rentals. Please inform the sales representative of your active duty or military status when you make your reservation.

Vets-Cars.com - An auto dealer association that pledges "thanks, respect, low up-front pricing, transparency and a superior showroom experience for U.S. Veterans, Active Duty and Family members.

Veterans Advantage - Membership is under $5 a month and provides access to thousands of discounts including Continental & United airlines, Amtrak, Wendy's, Footlocker, Dell, Greyhound, car rentals, Verizon and many other military discounts.

Veteran's Holiday's - Offers honorably discharged veteran's affordable condominium vacations at resorts around the world.

Verizon Wireless - Offers 15% on monthly plans costing $35 and above and 25% off accessories for all Federal Government Employees through its Consumer Accounts Department. Verizon Wireless offers three phones for free (CDM 180; PN-120 and LGVX3450). The service agreement can be one year or two years. The activation and shipping fees are waived. Family time plans (minimum 2 lines/maximum 5 lines per plan) pool the minutes together at$9.99 per phone add-on charge per month after the first two phones. Go to www.verizonwireless.com/discount and enter in your official military email address (personal email addresses cannot be accepted). Verizon wireless will send an email link and showing the discounted equipment and rates, as well as allow you to register an existing line of service for discounting. Also, you may contact Verizon Wireless at 1-800-922-0204.

Vettix - Submit a wish list for tickets. Vettix accepts tax deductible ticket donations from individuals and companies, then donates them to veterans for free through the Hero's Wish program. Other discounts are available as well.

Victory Motorcycles - Special offers vary but typically all Active and Retired Police and Firefighter Personnel are eligible for a discount. See the special offers section at www.victorymotorcycles.com

Walgreen's - 10 % off with a valid military ID card every Tuesday.

Walt Disney World Resort - Walt Disney World Resort offers U.S. military personnel four-day Military Promotional Tickets for just $138 each and up to 40 % off select Disney Resort Hotels

Wedding Ring Depot - Military members receive 10% off the purchase of wedding rings by using the code MILITARY at checkout.

White Flash Engagement Ring Discount - Active-Duty Armed Forces members receive 10% off engagement rings or diamonds. Enter promotional code "Military Discount" at checkout. Note: The website asks to send proof of military ID. It is against the law to send a photocopy or reproduction of a military ID.

Wicked Bride Stationary - Wicked Bride is proud to offer a military discount of 10% off the total order. (Proof of enlistment will be required.)

Wilson's Leather - Military personnel and their spouses get 10% off on clothes, accessories and other merchandise, in-store with military ID or call 1-866-305-4704.

Wendy's - Discount varies, simply ask and have a valid military ID card with you.

Wet Seal - 10 % military discount at www.wetseal.com

Whataburger - Discount varies, simply ask and have a valid military ID card with you.

World of Coca Cola - $2 off standard admission price for service members with ID, and up to 4 guests.

Wyndham Hotels - Discounts vary at 140 locations. And it also Depends on availability. Must present a valid military ID card upon check-in.

Zale's Diamond Store - Military members receive a 10% discount on any item that is not already discounted. In order to get the discount, you must call Zales to have it applied.

YMCA - YMCA centers that participate in the Military Outreach Initiative offer free and discounted memberships and child-care for military families.

Zaxby's - 10 % off with military ID.

Zoara - Military members receive a 10% discount on fine jewelry by registering with a valid military e-mail and entering the code USMILDISC at checkout.

www.bodybuilding.com - 10% discount
www.rei.com - up to 35% off new arrivals
www.carthartt.com -10% off for military
www.ace.com - 10% - 15% off (get 10% off $100 purchase / get 15% off $150+ purchase)
www.nflshop.com - 10% off for military
www.wine.com - 10% off for military
www.bluenile.com - 10% off for military
www.ticketnetwork.com - 5% off any ticket purchase
www.expedia.com - up to 5% off early bookings
www.kohls.com - 15% off $100+ purchase. Code: catch15off
www.sweetstayforsoldiers.com - exclusive discounts on top hotels and resorts for military
www.sandals.com - 10% off Caribbean vacations
www.cocacola.com - 20% off site wide
www.WylieWagg.com - 10% discount off an entire purchase for all active duty and retired U.S. Military; all that is required for the discount is a valid military ID.

All Federal employees are able to get a 15 % discount on their personal cell phones by calling their carrier and mentioning The Federal Telecommunications Act of 1996 – Discount to Federal Employees Past and Present. Military members must indicate supervisor's name, telephone number, and full address so that military status can be verified.

Nextel
Sprint
T – Mobile
Verizon

"To dilute the will to win is to destroy the purpose of the game. There is no substitute for victory." – Gen. Douglas Mac Arthur

What is your idea of Paradise? Perhaps it's digging your toes into warm, white sand and listening to the ocean's gentle rolling surf. It could be the exhilaration of nonstop activity and the promise of adventure at every turn. Or maybe, it's just taking a "time-out" from everyday life to just kick back and relax, recharge and reconnect with those you love.

Armed Forces Recreation Center (AFRC) resorts provide an array of affordable, wholesome vacation opportunities exclusively to the brave service members, and their families and other authorized patrons of the Total Defense Force. At AFRC resorts, they are focused on providing world-class service and assuring that their guests experience the vacation of a lifetime!

Whether it's strolling barefoot on the alabaster shores of Hawaii, or exploring medieval European castles, or discovering the enchantment of the Magic Kingdom, or exploring the exotic city of Seoul, your perfect paradise awaits.

Wilkommen im Bavaria

It's not just the altitude that will take your breath away. Whether you're seeking an intimate Bavarian dream vacation or high adventure, Edelweiss Lodge and Resort promises to peacefully surround you in Bavarian culture and luxury accommodations.

Edelweiss Lodge and Resort offers an array of guest amenities, including entertainment, and recreation activities. Enjoy a sightseeing tour or a day on the slopes; reap the benefits of a therapeutic massage, work out in the wellness club; take a dip in the indoor pool, or simply unwind in the outdoor hot tub. Relax in the restaurants featuring foods from around the world, including regional cuisine and all-American favorites.
And let's not forget:

- ➢ Majestic Alpine view
- ➢ Spacious guestrooms and cozy wood cabins
- ➢ Alpine adventures, recreation and guided tour.
- ➢ Spa services
- ➢ Full-service conference facility
- ➢ High-speed internet access

No matter what the season or the occasion, make it memorable. Make your vacation destination Edelweiss Lodge and Resort.

Reservation Information:

From Europe: (00-49) 8821-9440
From USA: (011-49) 8821-9440
Website: www.EdelweissLodgeandResort.com
Email: vacation@edelweisslodgeandresort.com

Hello Sunshine!

Go ahead. Pinch yourself. You're not dreaming. Experience the warm Florida sun, cascading waterfalls, lush tropical gardens, spectacular views, or a dip in the pool.

Not quite there yet? How about a visit to the enchanting **MAGIC KINGDOM** on Walt Disney World® Resort? This hot spot and other area attractions are just minutes away from Shades of Green on Walt Disney World® Resort. The guest services staff can assist you with discounted tickets for all area attractions and vacation planning.

Imagine a peaceful wooed setting surrounding 586 oversized guestrooms, cascading waterfalls, lush landscaped tropical gardens, spectacular views from private patios or balconies amid stunning sunrises. With diverse dining options, championship golf, plenty of kids' activities and a premier location on Walt Disney World® Resort, Shades of Green has all you are looking for in a totally relaxing vacation destination.

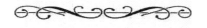

There's no shortage of options when you stay here. The swimming pools, including a children's pool and play area, exceptional dining, banquet, and meeting facilities satisfy a variety of needs.

An important part of any vacation is trying new restaurants. They offer a variety of dining options that will suit every taste. From family- casual to sophisticated, their specialty is serving you!

Within minutes to **MAGIC KINGDOM** and other **DISNEY** attractions; it has very spacious guestrooms, two heated swimming pools, a children's wading pool and play area, exceptional dining and high-speed internet access.

At Shades of Green, you've come to the right place for family fun and relaxation!

Reservation Information:

Website: www.shadesofgreen.org
Email: reservations@shadesofgreen.org

Aloha e Komo Mai!

Your tropical Hawaiian dream vacation awaits you at the Hale Koa Hotel. Diamond Head, the sparkling blue Pacific, lush landscaped tropical gardens, Polynesian entertainment, unsurpassed hospitality and more, are here for your vacation enjoyment. Whether you are strolling barefoot on the sand, sunbathing lazily on Waikiki Beach, or simply relaxing comfortably, you will simply be dazzled by this Polynesian paradise.

You can enjoy the Hawaiian sunsets while sipping their world-famous Mai Tai at the Barefoot Bar, or experience and enjoy the culinary delights at Koko's Café, Bibas, or the Hale Koa Room restaurants. The in-house entertainment features magic, songs and dances of Polynesia, and the luau on Waikiki Beach.

- Beach services rent surf and snorkel equipment
- Spa services
- Tennis courts
- Sand Volleyball
- Outdoor Racquetball courts

- World-Class golfing opportunities near the hotel
- Arrange tours of local attractions or take an outer island hop
- Military exchange, gift shops, jewelry, flower shop and sundries
- Enjoy a wide range of dining and entertainment on the property

Reservation Information:

Website: www.halekoa.com
Email: reservations@halekoa.com
1-800-367-6027 (CONUS)

Land of the Morning Calm

Ahn-yong-ha-o! Experience Asia in Style.

Welcome to the Land of the Morning Calm in Seoul, Korea. Supporting the Yongsan military community, the Dragon Hill Lodge has a myriad of services including a first-class fitness and health club, restaurants, lounges, and a specialty shopping mall. The hotel is a pleasant escape from the bustle and excitement of downtown Seoul.

Nestled in the heart of Seoul, Korea, the Dragon Hill Lodge is the gateway to Asia's mystical culture. Visit internationally acclaimed museums and art galleries, attend a lively sporting event, or simply enjoy world-class shopping!

Guests can relax in a number of restaurants and lounges or unwind in the state-of-the-art health club and pool. Additional amenities include a number of services such as the gift store, a flower shop, the tourism desk and a beauty salon. Premier conference rooms and lush landscaped gardens offer elegance and variety for business meetings or special events.

- o Within minutes of the exciting Seoul City Center
- o Premier conference rooms and gardens
- o Elegant and very comfortable guestrooms
- o Irresistible restaurants and comfortable lounges
- o Travel and Tour experts

Whether on vacation or on official travel, choose the Dragon Hill Lodge for a memorable lifetime experience!

Reservation Information:

Phone: (011-82-2) 7918-222 (24 hours)
Website: www.dragonhilllodge.com
Email: reservations@dhl.korea.army.mil

ROOMS WITH A VIEW PROGRAM

The great thing about camping is the seclusion and serenity. The bad thing is, well, you're camping. There's the whole sleeping on the ground business; except when you're lying awake wondering what's scratching outside the tent? Thanks to Rooms with a View cabin-rental program, visitors to Arizona's national forests can hit the backcountry and still enjoy a bed and other comforts of home.

Several years ago, the Forest Service began sprucing up historical cabins and renting them to the public. Lodgings range from a small adobe cottage in the Santa Rita Mountains to a stone cabin with a spectacular view of the San Francisco Peaks to a three-bedroom Art Deco ranch in the shadow of Cathedral Rock in Sedona, Arizona.

Just don't expect a mini-bar or turndown service. these are rustic retreats, each with a distinct character and limited amenities. Some have running water, indoor toilets and complete kitchens. Others aren't so plush. Make sure you check out all the information provided on the website provided for each cabin rental. If you are unable find what you are looking for, you can also call the telephone number that is provided.

U.S. Forest Service's Rooms with a View Program offers cabin rentals in some of the state's most beautiful places. These cabins are not mass-produced rentals. Each is unique and reflects the history and character of the place where it is located, all for not much more than you would pay for motel room in Phoenix. You should know that these are not luxury rentals.

If you want chocolates on your pillow, you will need to bring them yourself – along with sheets, toilet paper and, in some cases, an axe to cut your own firewood. Think camping, indoors. Each cabin has a past and a story to tell. And if it doesn't make you fall in love with Arizona all over again, just step outside.

Recreation.gov offers a military discount for U.S. Army Corps of Engineers facilities. Discount applies to Active military members and Department of Defense civilians who:

- are between tours of duty, **_or_**
- have returned from their tour of duty in a hostile fire zone
- can present a DD Form 2A or CAC Card to verify active member of U.S. Military

If you think you might qualify, this discount must be applied for by phone prior to placing your reservation. Contact 1-888-448-1474. Note: If sites are going quickly, you can process your reservation and then you can call in to apply for the waiver.

America the Beautiful Senior Pass, America the Beautiful-The National Parks and Federal Recreational Lands Pass Series, America the Beautiful Access Pass are all good for discounts on cabin rentals.

Kent Springs Cabin

The fireplace is charming, the dual living rooms are quirky, and the expansive deck overlooking Daniels Creek is impressive. But what makes this stone and wood cabin in the Santa Rita Mountains south of Tucson memorable is the way it takes the surrounding oak and juniper woodland, literally, with boulders and a juniper tree built right into the structure. Ben and Anne Daniels homesteaded the area around 1910. A former Rough Rider, Ben owned one of the dozen or so mines that operated Madera Canyon in the early 1900's. He was elected Pima County Sheriff in 1920.

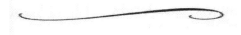

Annie served as the county's school superintendent. The remains of their original cabin is nearby. The current structure grew up around the landscape, beginning in the early 1950's. It expanded to include a bathroom, a porch, a dining room and an additional living room in the 60's and 70's.

The Friends of Madera Canyon renovated the cabin in the 1990's. The cabin is located in scenic Madera Canyon, 15 miles east of Green Valley, AZ, and within 1 hour of Tucson. The cabin can accommodate up to 8 people.

You can call the Ranger Station listed below for information or log on to the website below to find out more information.

Nogales Ranger District
520-281-2296
1-877-444-6777
www.recreation.gov

Caldwell Cabin

Imagine, a cabin nestled amongst the tall ponderosa pine trees. Now, ease back in an Adirondack chair on the front porch and soak in the panorama of a long, grassy meadow ringed with pines. And is that a herd of grazing elk?

Probably. Wildlife aplenty in these mountains, including the re-introduced Mexican grey wolf. As the cabin sits at 7,600 feet, the fireplace proves most welcome. Because of the high elevation, summer temperatures are pleasant and cool, providing a nice respite from the heat of lower deserts.

The cabin allows up to 6 visitors to step back in time to a more rustic and historic era in eastern Arizona. Originally constructed in the 1920's, it was a one room homestead. Expanded around 1940, to include a bathroom, a small bedroom and living room with a fireplace. It is located approximately 30 miles southwest of the town of Alpine in beautiful White Mountains. Some of the roads are gravel.

You can call the Ranger Station listed below for information or log on to the website below to find out more information.

Alpine Ranger District
928-339-5000
1-877-444-6777
www.recreation.gov

Kendrick Cabin

Kendrick Cabin perfectly reflects its former life as a seasonal fireguard station. The rustic, three-bedroom masonry and wood cabin are a retired U.S. Forest Service fire guard station constructed in the 1960's. Don't be surprised to hear elk bugle or catch a glimpse of a pronghorn. It lies just minutes from downtown Flagstaff, AZ and about an hour from Grand Canyon National Park. The cabin sits in the lap of San Francisco Peaks, with wraparound high-country views. At 7,900 feet, be prepared for some blissfully cool days and cozy nights by the wood-burning stove and enjoy the peace and solitude.

The cabin can accommodate up to 10 people and give them the chance to experience spectacular mountain views as well as numerous hiking and mountain biking trails. Located just a short 22 miles north of Flagstaff, the area is home to elk, deer, antelope, fox, coyotes, mountain lions, numerous birds and other animals.

You can call the Ranger Station listed below for information or log on to the website below to find out more information.

Coconino Forest Ranger District
928-526-0866
1-877-444-6777
www.recreation.gov

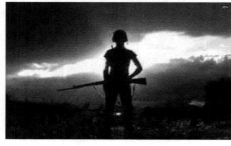

Kentucky Camp

This is the only cabin where you stay in town. A ghost town, to be sure, but that's part of the rich experience. Kentucky Camp was built in 1904 as a gold-mining venture and abandoned in 1912 after the mine engineer mysteriously plunged to his death from the window of a Tucson hotel. A handful of buildings served as headquarters for the Santa Rita Mining Company from 1902 to1906. It also served as a cattle ranch in the 1960's.

The Forest Service acquired the land in 1989 and it has since become an ideal location for guests seeking a unique lodging experience, rich in mining and ranching history. Spanning four life zones and several ecosystems between desert and mountain peaks, the area surrounding the camp and cabin is considered a 'sky-island, supporting abundant and biologically diverse plant and animal communities.

Now all that remains are a cabin and a headquarters building. The cabin can accommodate up to 5 people.

The headquarters building is a day use area only and can accommodate up to 50 people Available for weddings, meetings, retreats and family reunions. Located in the Santa Rita Mountains, 9 miles north of Sonoita, AZ.

You can call the Ranger Station listed below for information or log on to the website below to find out more information.

Kentucky Camp Cabin and Headquarters Building
520-281-2296
1-877-444-6777
www.recreation.gov

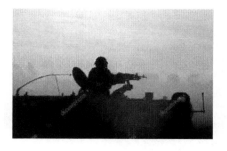

Fernow Cabin

If you're having trouble deciding between pine forests and red-rock country, this rustic cabin tucked in a scenic draw atop the Mongollon Rim gives you both. It's hidden high in the pines but has views and trails leading deep into the Red Rock-Seret Mountain Wilderness Area. This rustic 3-bedroom log cabin is a retired U.S. Forest Service guard station constructed in the 1970's to house firefighters during fire season. Nestled in a beautiful ponderosa pine setting, the cabin is isolated which provides privacy with great opportunities for getting back to nature. This quaint, forested retreat near Flagstaff, AZ and Sedona, AZ, can accommodate up to 8 people. The cabin is adjacent to the Sycamore Canyon and Red Rock-Secret Mountain Wilderness Areas, which boasts numerous hiking trails.

You can call the Ranger Station listed below for information or log on to the website below to find out more information.

Coconino Forest Ranger District
928-526-0866
1-877-444-6777
www.recreation.gov

Apache Maid Cabin

Originally constructed in 1909 by Charles Babbitt and William Dickinson as a ranch house for cattlemen, then later used as a U.S. Forest Service Ranger Station. The cabin is surrounded by the shade of a ponderosa pine forest and is just south of the Mongollon Rim. It sits at 6,382 feet and has summers that are characteristically sunny, warm and dry, with the occasional afternoon thunderstorm. This little rustic Forest Service facility is located at the eastern base of Apache Maid Mountain. Can accommodate up to 6 people. It is located 2 hours north of Phoenix, AZ; 45 minutes north of Camp Verde, AZ.

You can call the Ranger Station listed below for information or log on to the website below to find out more information.

Coconino Forest Ranger District
928-526-0866
1-877-444-6777 / www.recreation.gov

Spring Valley Cabin

Enjoy spectacular views, cross-country ski trails, and time "away from it all" at this 90-year-old cabin and bunkhouse that sits at the wind-brushed edge of an alpine meadow, with vistas stretching to the San Francisco Peaks. You'll feel fortunate to have a yard that extends to the horizon. Just don't get so overprotective that you tell the grazing mule deer and pronghorns to get off your lawn.

Spring Valley Cabin and Bunkhouse offers a peaceful retreat with spectacular views, quiet solitude, wildlife viewing opportunities and access to cross-country ski trails, all at just minutes away from Flagstaff, AZ, and one hour from Grand Canyon National Park.

Located at 7,320 feet, overlooking a wide meadow while being nestled beneath mature ponderosa pines with views of Kendrick Peak and nearby trails lined with oaks, aspens, pines, firs and spruce create a fall backdrop for long walks or rides. The cabin was constructed in 1917 as the residence for rangers who worked at the guard station.

The bunkhouse served as the office. It is still occasionally used as a field station for U.S. Forest Service employees.

Winter brings a mix of sun with cold temperatures and occasional winter storms. Summer temperatures are relatively pleasant, but weather can be unpredictable. This year –round getaway can host up to 14 people between the cabin and bunkhouse.

You can call the Ranger Station listed below for information or log on to the website below to find out more information.

Williams Ranger District
928-635-5600
1-877-444-6777
www.recreation.gov

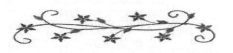

Portal Bunkhouse and Portal CCC House

The Portal Bunkhouse is a two-room cabin and the Portal CCC House is a 5-room cabin located one mile west of Portal, AZ. Two of the Forest Service's newest cabin rentals that occupy prime real estate in Cave Creek Canyon, a premier birding destination and an area of uncommon beauty, with dramatic rhyolite cliffs rising high above a leafy canopy of oaks and sycamores. The canyon's soaring cliffs, with their caves and pinnacles, are often described as "Arizona's 'Secret' Grand Canyon".

Built in1933 and listed on the National Register of Historic Places, the Portal Bunkhouse is one of the few remaining structures from the Civilian Conservation Corps camp that was located here, and it's one of the era's finest examples of river-cobblestone masonry. The nearby CCC House is located at the entrance to Cave Creek Canyon at an elevation of 5,000 feet. It first served as the camp's garage, then as housing for a telephone operator and switchboard. The Bunkhouse can sleep up to 4 people and the CCC House can sleep up to 5 people.

You can call the Ranger Station listed below for information or log on to the website below to find out more information.

Coronado Ranger District
520-364-3468
1-877-444-6777
www.recreation.gov

Half Moon Ranch

Half Moon Ranch is a ranch style house located in the east Cochise Stronghold in the Dragoon Mountains of the Coronado National Forest. The house is situated in a dramatic canyon that provides excellent hiking, mountain biking, and horseback riding opportunities. Surrounded by the rugged beauty of the Cochise Stronghold, at an elevation of 5,000 feet. This sparsely wooded area is a protective rampart of granite spires, sheer cliffs, balanced rocks and boulders which were once the refuge of Apache Chief Cochise. The house lies in a mountain range or 'sky-island' in the Coronado National Forest, rising dramatically from the desert floor, supporting abundant and biologically diverse plant and animal communities. The house can comfortably accommodate up to 10 people.

You can call the Ranger Station listed below for information or log on to the website below to find out more information.

Coronado Ranger District
520-364-3468
1-877-444-6777
www.recreation.gov

Crescent Moon Ranch

You won't find utter isolation at this Sedona cabin, but you will have Cathedral Rock (one of the most photographed scenes in the Southwest), rising just beyond your back porch, like the most awesome lawn ornament ever imagined. Walk out your door to Oak Creek and a sweet swimming hole complete with a rope swing.

Crescent Moon Ranch is an exceptional year-round place to stay in beautiful Sedona, AZ. Placed beside a tree-lined creek with Sedona's famous red rock cliffs in the background. Its location offers a serene natural setting. The site lies in the high desert at the base of the Mogollon Rim, a 200-mile slope that ranges between 5,000 and 7,000 feet in elevation. Crescent Moon Ranch was built by ranchers of the original homestead at an elevation of 4,000 feet, the cabin was later made available for public use by the U.S. Forest Service.

You can call the Ranger Station listed below for information or log on to the website below to find out more information.

Coconino Forest Ranger District
928-526-0866
1-877-444-6777
www.recreation.gov

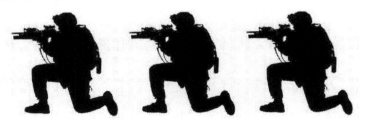

Hull Cabin

The cabin sits in a secluded meadow surrounded by a strand of old growth ponderosa pine trees, at an elevation of 6,500 feet. The cabin was originally a one-room homestead, constructed by the Hull family in the late 1880's with hand hewn logs as part of a sheep ranch. and then was acquired by the Forest Service in 1907 for use as a ranger station. Located just one mile south of Grand Canyon National Park, Hull Cabin is the oldest surviving historic cabin near the Grand Canyon's south rim. The location provides easy access to Grandview Lookout Tower, which offers 360-degree views of the canyon and surrounding forest. Summer temperatures on the South Rim are relatively pleasant, but weather can be unpredictable. The cabin can sleep up to 6 people.

You can call the Ranger Station listed below for information or log on to the website below to find out more information.

Kaibab Forest Ranger District
928-638-2443
1-877-444-6777
www.recreation.gov

Horsethief Basin Cabin

The original cabin was built in 1939 as quarters and a staging area for Forest Service crews in charge of protecting the southern end of the Bradshaw Mountains against wildfires. The cabin was remodeled and modernized over the years, but eventually fell into disuse by the 1980's. Now, the cabin enjoys a second life as a rental cabin for the Forest Service.

Anglers will appreciate the short stroll to Horsethief Basin Lake, stocked with largemouth bass, channel catfish and sunfish, and offering non-motorized boating. But there's no reason for hikers to feel left out, with trails leading to Horsethief Canyon, Twin Peaks, Castle Creek and Jim Creek. Horsethief Cabin is nestled in the Bradshaw Mountains near Horsethief Basin Lake and Castle Creek Wilderness Area in Prescott National Forest. Situated in a clearing of ponderosa pines at an elevation of over 6,000 feet in the Bradshaw Mountains of the Prescott National Forest.

The area is rich in history, including early Native American inhabitants and later in the 1860's, home to horse thieves and rustled livestock. The cabin can accommodate up to 6 people comfortably. Dense populations of mule deer and javelina inhabit the area, along with a few mountain lions, bobcats, black bears, coyotes, rabbits, foxes, skunks, and badgers.

You can call the Ranger Station listed below for information or log on to the website below to find out more information.

Prescott Forest Ranger District
928-443-8000
1-877-444-6777
www.recreation.gov

The Shaw House

The Shaw House is a stone cabin located in the east Cochise Stronghold in the Dragoon Mountains of the Coronado National Forest. The house is nestled in a dramatic landscape of canyons, rock formations, and the shade of several large cottonwood trees, offering guests a unique lodging experience which is surrounded by the rugged beauty of the Cochise Stronghold in the Coronado National Forest. This sparsely wooded area is a protective rampart of granite spires, sheer cliffs, balanced rocks and boulders, which were once the refuge for Apache Chief Cochise.

The area is abundant with wildlife, including white-tailed deer and mule deer, rabbits, wild turkeys, and squirrels. Bats, black bear, Coati, foxes, ring-tailed cats, bobcats, and mountain lion find habitat in the area as well, but are more often seen in the twilight and nocturnal hours.

The Shaw House is an 8-room house and can sleep up to 10 people.

You can call the Ranger Station listed below for information or log on to the website below to find out more information.

Coronado Ranger District
520-364-3468
1-877-444-6777
www.recreation.gov

Sycamore Cabin

In 1938, the Civilian Conservation Corps constructed the cabin, which served as a residence for the district ranger and later became housing for fire crews during fire season. The cabin is located at an elevation of 4,000 feet and sits on the banks of Sycamore Creek which runs directly behind the cabin and is canopied by cottonwoods and Arizona sycamores. A section of the Great Western Trail, part of a nearly 4,500-mile corridor stretching from Mexico to Canada, curves past the cabin.

Sycamore cabin provides a unique recreation opportunity and lodging experience. The cabin's capacity is up to 8 people, however sleeping accommodations within the cabin are for 6. Today, the cabin is available for reservation year-round for guests seeking relaxation and recreation in central Arizona.

Located at an elevation of 4,000 feet and sits on the edge of Sycamore Creek, providing an opportunity to explore a unique riparian area just outside the back door. Dense populations of mule deer and javelina inhabit this area, along with a few mountain lions, bobcats, black bears, coyotes, rabbits, foxes, skunks, and badgers. Enjoy the serenity, spectacular views, local hiking trails, the Great Western Trail, and time "away from it all."

You can call the Ranger Station listed below for information or log on to the website below to find out more information.

Prescott Forest Ranger District
928-443-8000
1-877-444-6777
www.recreation.gov

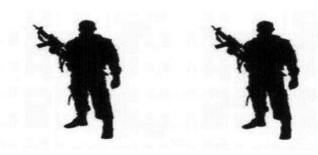

Palisades Ranger Residence Cabin

The Palisades Ranger Residence Cabin is located within the Palisades Administrative Site in the Santa Catalina Mountains, 20 miles northwest of Tucson, AZ. It is reached via the Sky Island Scenic Byway, a historic, scenic, and ecological drive from the Sonoran Desert to the dense forests at 8,000 feet elevation. Approximately one hour from Tucson and provides terrific access to a myriad of recreational opportunities, including hiking, birding, horseback riding, picnicking, sightseeing and visiting historic areas. The cabin lies in a mountain range or" sky-island" in the Coronado National Forest, rising dramatically from the desert floor, supporting abundant and biologically diverse plant and animal communities. From the desert floor to the upper slopes of Mt. Lemmon, life zones vary from Sonoran Desert to sub alpine forest. The cabin can accommodate up to 4 people.

You can call the Ranger Station listed below for information or log on to the website below to find out more information.

Coronado Ranger District
520-364-3468
520-749-8700
1-877-444-6777
www.recreation.gov

Arizona Resorts that offer a Military Discount

Arizona Golf Resort Hotel
425 South Power Road
Mesa, AZ 85206
480-832-3202
www.arizonagolfresort.com

Arizona Golf Resort Hotel offers a military discount that is based on availability and season. You must call and ask for their military/ government rate. Special rate includes a free breakfast every day of your stay.

Arizona Grand Resort

8000 South Arizona Grand Parkway
Phoenix, AZ 85044
Reservations: 602-438-9000
Toll Free: 1-877-800-4888
www.arizonagrandresort.com

Arizona Grand Resort offers a military discount that is based on availability. The discount is easier to get by calling rather than booking online. You must provide a valid military ID when you check-in.

Amara Resort Hotel and Spa

100 Amara Lane
Sedona, AZ 85336
928-282-4828
www.amararesort.com
www.kimptonhotels.com

Amara Resort and Spa offers a government/military discount that is based on availability and black-out dates. Check their website(s) for more information. You must show a valid military ID card when you check-in.

Bell Rock Inn

6246 State Route 179
Sedona, AZ 86351
1-866-599-6674
1-888-950-5062
1-844-854-8682
www.diamondresorts.com

Bell Rock Inn offers a military discount available seven days a week and is based on availability. Rate is refundable. You can call the resort for details or you can book online. You must show a valid military ID card when you check-in.

Cabins on Strawberry Hill

5306 North Highway 87
Pine, AZ 85544
928-476-4252
www.azcabins.com

Cabins on Strawberry Hill does not offer an 'official' discount. But they will offer military and veterans discounts anytime Sunday through Thursday, excluding holidays. Must show a valid military ID card at check-in.

Camelback Inn, a JW Marriott Resort and Spa

5402 East Lincoln Drive
Scottsdale, AZ 85253
480-948-1700
www.marriott.com/scottsdale-camelback-inn-and-spa

Marriott offers a government rate for active duty military, civilian federal employees. You may check the availability of rooms offered at government discount rates by using the Marriott.com website. Must show a valid military ID.

Canyon Ranch

8600 East Rockcliff Road
Tucson, AZ 85750
520-749-9000
www.canyonranch.com

Canyon Ranch does not offer a military discount, but they do offer a 25% discount if you are an Arizona resident. Check their website for rates and for more information.

Carefree Resort and Conference Center

37220 Mule Train Road
Carefree, AZ 85377
1-888-692-4343
www.carefree-resort.com

The Carefree Resort offers a 10% discount or their BAR rate for military and veterans. Must show a valid military ID card at check-in.

Casino Del Sol Resort
5655 West Velencia Road
Tucson, AZ 85757
1-855-765-7829
www.casinodelsolresort.com

Casino Del Sol Resort usually offers a10% discount for military and veterans, when available. You must show a valid military ID card at check-in.

CopperWynd Resort and Club
13225 North Eagle Ridge Drive
Fountain Hills, AZ 85268
480-333-1900
www.copperwynd.com

CopperWynd Resort and Club offers a government/military rate that is about 15% off the normal rate. They will offer the same rate for retired veterans as well, if rooms are available. You can only call to make your reservation, let them know you are military (or government employee) so you can get this special rate. You must show a valid military ID when you check-in.

Crowne Plaza San Marcos Golf Resort
1 North San Marcos Place
Chandler, AZ 85225
480-812-9000
www.ihg.com
www.sanmarcosresort.com

Crowne Plaza San Marcos Golf Resort offers a government rate. If calling for reservations, just ask for the government discount, or if you are booking online, use the rate drop down selector and highlight government rate. Just be ready to show your military ID card when you check-in.

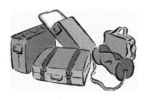

116

JW Marriott Desert Ridge Resort and Spa

5350 East Marriott Drive
Phoenix, AZ 85054
480-293-5000
1-800-835-6206 for Reservations
www.marriott.com

Marriott offers a government rate for active duty military, civilian federal employees. You may check the availability of rooms offered at government discount rates by using the Marriott.com website. Must show a valid military ID.

Embassy Suites Biltmore

2630 East Camelback Road
Phoenix, AZ 85016
602-955-3992
www.embassysuites3.hilton.com

Hilton Hotels and Resorts offer a 10% discount off leisure stays for active duty and retired military and their families at participating locations. You just need to show a valid military ID card.

Esplendor Resort at Rio Rico

1069 Camino Caralampi
Rio Rico, AZ 85648
520-281-1901
www.esplendor-resort.com

Esplendor Resort offers a military / veteran's discount. You must call to check the amount of the discount. Discount is based on availability. You must show a valid military ID when you check-in.

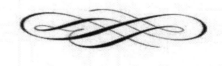

Fairfield Sedona Resort

1500 Kestral Circle
Sedona, AZ 86336
www.dreamsedona.com/fairfield-sedona-resort-html
www.diamondresorts.com

The resort offers a military discount available seven days a week and is based on availability. Rate is refundable. You can call the resort for details or you can book online. You must show a valid military ID card when you check-in.

Firesky Resort and Spa-A Kimpton Hotel

4925 North Scottsdale Road
Scottsdale, AZ 85251
480-945-7666
www.fireskyresort.com

Firesky Resort and Spa offers government per-diem rates. We roll out the red carpet for government and military personnel, offering an exceptional destination and stylish accommodations at special rates to make per diem travel comfortable, fun and easy.

Francisco Grande Hotel and Golf Resort

12684 West Gila Bend Highway
Casa Grande, AZ 85193
520-836-6444
1-800-237-4238

The Francisco Grande Hotel and Golf Resort offers a government rate from April through December. Must show a valid military ID card at check-in.

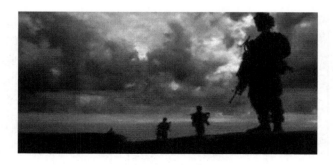

Gold Canyon Golf Resort

6100 South Kings Ranch Road
Gold Canyon, AZ 85118
480-982-9090
1-800-827-5281 Toll Free
www.gcgr.com

Gold Canyon Golf Resort offers a military discount that is equivalent to the AAA rate. Discount is based on availability and demand. You can call in your reservation or you can book one online. Just let them know that you are military, and they will adjust the rate for you. You must show a valid military ID when you check-in.

Grand Canyon Railway and Hotel

233 North Grand Canyon Blvd.
Williams, AZ 86046
928-635-4010
1-800-843-8724
www.thetrain.com

The Grand Canyon Railway and Resort offers a 15% military /veterans discount on train reservations and a 15% military /veterans discount on hotel reservations. You will need to call the number above to make reservations. You must show a valid military ID card when you check-in.

Greer Lodge Resort and Cabins

80 Main Street
Greer, AZ 85927
928-225-7620
www.greerlodgeaz.com

Greer Lodge Resort and Cabins offers a 10% discount for military. Discount is based on availability. You can call in your reservation or book one online. You must show a valid military ID when you check-in.

Hacienda Del Sol Guest Ranch Resort

5501 North Hacienda Del Sol Road
Tucson, AZ 85718
520-299-1501
1-800-728-6514 Toll Free
www.haciendadelsolresort.com

The Hacienda Del Sol Guest Ranch Resort offers a military and veterans discount Sunday through Thursday and based on availability. You can call in your reservation or book on online. Just make sure you ask for the discount. You must show a valid military ID when you check-in.

Havasu Dunes Resort

620 South Lake Havasu Avenue
Lake Havasu, AZ 86406
Reservations: 1-866-921-5136
www.extraholidays.com

Havasu Dunes Resort offers a 10% military discount for active duty and retired military. For more information, call the reservations number 1-866-921-5136 and ask for their military discount. Must show a valid military ID card when you check-in.

Hilton Tucson El Conquistador Golf and Tennis Resort

10000 North Oracle Road
Tucson, AZ 85704
520-544-5000
1-800-HILTON
   (44-5866)
www.hiltonelconquistador.com
www.hilton.com

Hilton Hotels and Resorts offer a military rate for leisure stays for active duty and retired military and their families at participating locations. The military rate varies by occupancy and season. You can go online at either of the websites above and get the military rate there as well. You just need to show a valid military ID card when you check-in.

Hyatt Regency Scottsdale Resort and Spa at Gainey Ranch

7500 East Doubletree Ranch Road
Scottsdale, AZ 85258
480-444-1234 Central Reservation
904-588-1234 Hotel Reservations
www.scottsdale.hyatt.com

Hyatt Regency Scottsdale Resort and Spa at Gainey Ranch offers a government per diem rate that is good for government employees and active duty military on official business. You can call in your reservation or you can book one online. You must show proof of your active duty/official business status and you need to show a valid military ID when you check-in.

Hilton Scottsdale Resort and Villas

6333 North Scottsdale Road
Scottsdale, AZ 85250
480-948-7750
www.3.hilton.com
www.3.hilton.com/en/hotels/arizona/hilton-scottsdale
-resort-and-villas-SCTSHHF/index.html

Hilton Hotels and Resorts offer a 10% discount off leisure stays for active duty and retired military and their families at participating locations. You just need to show a valid military ID card.

Hilton Sedona at Bell Rock

90 Trail Drive
Sedona, AZ 86351
928-284-6940
1-877-2REDROCK
        (73-3762)
www.3.hilton.com
www.hiltonsedonaresort.com

Hilton Hotels and Resorts offer a 10% discount off leisure stays for active duty and retired military and their families at participating locations. You just need to show a valid military ID card.

Hassayampa Inn

122 East Gurley Street
Prescott, AZ 86301
928-778-9434
www.hassayampainn.com

The Hassayampa Inn offers a 10% discount for military and veterans Sunday through Thursday and if they can, depending on availability, on weekends. You can call in your reservation or you can book one online. You must show a valid military ID when you check-in.

Legacy Golf Resort

6808 South 32nd Street
Phoenix, AZ 85042
602-305-5500
Reservations: 1-866-859-5842
www.extendedholidays.com

Legacy Golf Resort offers a 10% military discount for active duty and retired military. For more information, call the reservations number 1-866-859-5842 or 602-305-5500 and ask for their military discount. Must show a valid military ID card when you check-in.

Loews Ventana Canyon Resort

7000 North Resort Drive
Tucson, AZ 85750
520-299-2020
1-800-234-5117 Reservations
www.loewshotels.com
www.loewshotels.com/ventana-canyon

Loews Hotels offer a military discount. Discount varies by occupancy and season. You can call their Reservations number 1-800-234-5117 and ask for the government rate or you can get the government rate online at www.loewshotels.com.

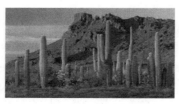

122

Lake Mohave Resort at Katherine's Landing

2690 East Katherine Spur Road
Katherine's Landing on Lake Mohave
Bullhead City, AZ 85929
928-754-3245
www.sevencrown.com

Lake Mohave Resort at Katherine's Landing offers a military discount on their boat rentals. You just have to ask for it and have a valid military ID card.

Los Abrigados Resort and Spa

160 Portal Lane
Sedona, AZ 86336
1-877-784-6835
1-800-438-2929 Reservations
www.losabridgadossedonaresort.com
www.diamondresorts.com

The resort offers a military discount available 7 days a week and is based on availability. Rate is refundable. You can call the resort for details or you can book online. Must show a valid military ID when you check-in.

Marriott Camelback Inn Resort Golf Club and Spa

5402 East Lincoln Drive
Scottsdale, AZ 85253
480-948-1700
www.marriott.com

Marriott offers a government rate for active duty military, civilian and federal employees. You may check the availability of rooms offered at government discount rates by using the Marriott.com website. Must show a valid military ID.

Marriott at McDowell Mountain

16770 North Perimeter Drive
Scottsdale, AZ 85260
480-502-3836
www.marriott.com

Marriott offers a government rate for active duty military, civilian federal employees. You may check the availability of rooms offered at government discount rates by using the Marriott.com website. Must show a valid military ID.

Millennium Resort, Scottsdale at McCormick Ranch

7401 North Scottsdale Road
Scottsdale, AZ 85253
1-800-243-1322
www.millenniumhotels.com/usa/millenniumscottsdale

As a salute to those serving our country in the capacity of either active duty military or government employee, Millennium hotels across North America are proud to offer special hotel rates. You must show a valid military ID or government ID when you check-in.

Omni Tucson National Golf Resort and Spa

2727 West Club Drive
Tucson, AZ 85742
520-247-2271
www.omnihotels.com

The Omni Tucson National Resort offers a military and veteran discount. All you have to do is call their reservations number 520-247-2271 and ask for the discount. Must provide a valid military ID when you check in.

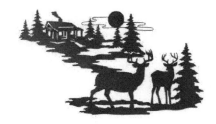

Omni Scottsdale Resort and Spa at Montelucia

4949 E. Lincoln Drive
Scottsdale, AZ 85253
480-627-3200
www.omnihotels.com

The Omni Scottsdale Resort and Spa at Montelucia offers a military and veteran discount. All you have to do is call their reservations number 480-627-3200 and ask for the discount. Must provide a valid military ID when you check-in.

Orange Tree Golf Resort

10601 North 56th Street
Scottsdale, AZ 85254
480-948-6100
1-866-859-5842 Toll Free
www.shellhospitality.com
www.extraholidays.com

The Orange Tree Golf Resort offers a 15% off for military and for retired military. Just need to show a valid military ID card.

Paradise Valley Double Tree Resort

5401 North Scottsdale Road
Scottsdale, AZ 85250
480-947-5400
www.doubletree.3.hilton.com

Hilton Hotels and Resorts offer a 10% discount off leisure stays for active duty and retired military and their families at participating locations. You just need to show a valid military ID card.

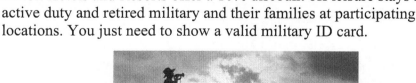
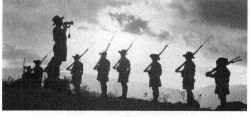

Phoenix Marriott Tempe at the Buttes

2000 West Westcourt Way
Tempe, AZ 85282
602-225-9000
www.marriott.com/hotels/travel/phxtm-phoenix
-mariott-tempe-at-the-buttes

Marriott offers a government rate for active duty military, civilian federal employees. You may check the availability of rooms offered at government discount rates by using the Marriott.com website. Must show a valid military ID.

Poco Diablo Resort

1752 State Route 179
Sedona, AZ 86336
928-282-7333
www.pocodiablo.com
www.diamondresorts.com

The Radisson Poco Diablo Resort offers a military rate that is based on availability. Discount is available seven days a week. With special rate, you also receive a $30 food voucher per day of your stay that you can use at the resort restaurant. You must call the resort and make a reservation, or you can book it online at one of the websites listed above. Must provide a valid military ID card when you check-in.

Pointe Hilton Squaw Peak

7677 North 16th Street
Phoenix, AZ 85020
602-997-2626
www.squawpeakhilton.com

Hilton Hotels and Resorts offer a 10% discount off leisure stays for active duty and retired military and their families at participating locations. You just need to show a valid military ID card.

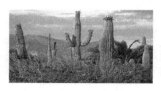

Pointe Hilton Tapatio Cliffs

11111 North 7th Street
Phoenix, AZ 85020
602-866-7500
www.tapatiocliffshilton.com

Hilton Hotels and Resorts offer a 10% discount off leisure stays for active duty and retired military and their families at participating locations. You just need to show a valid military ID card.

Rancho De Los Caballeros

1551 South Vulture Mine Road
Wickenburg, AZ 85390
928-684-5484
www.ranchodeloscaballeros.com

Rancho De Los Caballeros offers a special rate for military - The Full American Plan a very nice comfortable room and includes 3 meals per day per person. The cost for this American Plan is $160/night, plus 15% gratuity and 7.3% sales tax. You can call in your reservation or you can book one online. You must show a valid military ID when you check-in.

Red Agave Adventure Resort

120 Canyon Circle Drive
Sedona, AZ 86351
928-284-9327
1-877-284-9237 toll free
www.redagaveresort.net

The Red Agave offers a 10% military discount, 7 days a week. You can call in your reservation or book one online. You must show a valid military ID when you check-in.

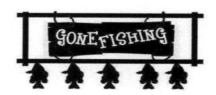

127

Ridge on Sedona Golf Resort

55 Sunridge Circle
Sedona, AZ 86351
928-284-9355
1-800-438-2929 Reservations
www.sedonagolfresort.com
www.diamondresorts.com

The resort offers a military discount available seven days a week and is based on availability. Rate is refundable. You can call the resort for details or you can book online. You must show a valid military ID card when you check-in.

Scottsdale Resort and Athletic Club

8235 East Indian Bend Road
Scottsdale, AZ 85250
480-344-0600
1-877-343-0033
www.scottsdaleresortandathleticclub.com

The Scottsdale Resort Club offers a 15% military discount for active duty ONLY. You must show a valid military ID and proof of being on active duty when you check-in.

Sedona Summit Resort

4055 Navoti Drive
Sedona, AZ 86336
1-866-844-0460
1-800-438-2929 Reservations
www.sedonasummitresort.com
www.diamondresorts.com

The resort offers a military discount available seven days a week and is based on availability. Rate is refundable. You can call the resort for details or you can book online. You must show a valid military ID card when you check-in.

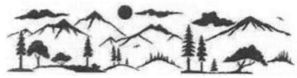

Smoke Tree Resort and Bungalows

7101 East Lincoln Drive
Paradise Valley, AZ 85253
480-948-7660
1-877-948-7660
www.smoketreeresoert.com

The Smoketree Resort and Bungalows offers $5.00 off the already promotional rate that is shown on their website for the military. You must show a valid military ID when you check-in.

JW Marriott Starr Pass Resort and Spa

3800 West Starr Pass Blvd.
Tucson, AZ 85745
1-888-236-2427 Reservations
1-800-721-7033 Customer Support
520-792-3500
www.marriott.com/hotels/travel/tussp-jw-marriott
-tucson-starr-pass-resort-and-spa
www.marriott.com

Marriott offers a government rate for active duty military, civilian federal employees. You may check the availability of rooms offered at government discount rates by using the Marriott.com website. Must show a valid military ID.

Scottsdale Links Resort

16858 North Perimeter Drive
Scottsdale, AZ 85260
480-563-0500
1-800-438-2929 for reservations
www.scottsdalelinksresort.com
www.diamondresorts.com

The Scottsdale Links Resort offers a discount for active duty military ONLY. You can call in your reservation or you can book one online. You must show a valid military ID when you check-in.

Talking Stick Resort

9800 East Indian Bend Road
Scottsdale, AZ 85256
480-850-7777 Resort
1-866-877-9897 Reservations
www.talkingstickresort.com

The Talking Stick resort offers a special military rate Sunday through Thursday if occupancy allows. You can call in your reservation or book one online. You must show a valid military ID when you check-in.

Temple Bar Resort

1 Main Street
Temple Bar Marina, AZ 86443
928-767-3211
www.templebarlakemead.com

Active Military, Veterans, Firefighters, Police and EMT's (Emergency Medical Technicians) of the United States are now eligible to receive a $200 discount off their houseboat rental and/or a 19% discount off powerboats, personal watercraft and other small boats. To receive this discount (credit before taxes), the renter must present valid documentation upon arrival and check-in. (Not required to be the primary name on the invoice).

- Any houseboat model in our fleet
- Any Forever Marina
- Any time
- No blackout dates

Cannot be combined with any other specials or offers. All other Houseboat Rental Terms and Conditions apply.

The Boulders

34631 North Tom Darlington Drive
Carefree, AZ 85377
480-488-9009 Resort
1-888-579-2631 Reservations
www.theboulders.com

The Boulders Resort and Spa offers a government rate for the military. Rate is based on availability and depends on the time that you want to stay. You can call in your reservation or you can book one online. When calling in, just ask for the government rate. You must show a valid military ID when you check-in.

The Fairmont Scottsdale Princess

7575 East Princess Drive
Scottsdale, AZ 85255
480-505-4848
www.scottsdaleprincess.com

The Fairmont Scottsdale Princess offers a military for active duty military. Just ask for the discount when book for your reservation. You must show a valid military ID card at check-in.

The Hermosa Inn

5532 North Palo Cristi Road
Paradise Valley, AZ 85253
602-955-8614
www.hermosainn.com

The Hermosa Inn offers a 10% discount for AAA Members and will be happy to extend this discount to military and veterans. Must show a valid military ID card at check-in.

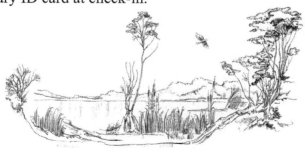

The Inn at Eagle Mountain

9800 North Summer Hill Blvd.
Fountain Hills, AZ 85268
480-816-3000
1-855-988-4745
www.innateaglemountain.com

The Inn at Eagle Mountain offers a 15% discount off the current room rate for military and veterans. They also offer a government per diem rate for government employees and active duty military. You can only call in your reservation You must show a valid military ID card at check-in.

The Lodge at Ventana Canyon

6200 North Club House Lane
Tucson, AZ 85750
520-577-1400
1-800-838-5701 - Toll Free
www.thelodgeatventanacanyon.com

The Lodge at Ventana Canyon offers a 10% discount off the current advertised room rate. Discount is based on availability. You can call in your reservation or you can book online. You must show a valid military ID when you check-in.

The Westin La Paloma Resort and Spa

3800 East Sunrise Drive
Tucson, AZ 85718
520-742-6000
www.westinlapalomaresort.com
www.starwoodhotels.com

The Westin La Paloma Resort and Spa offers a military rate, which varies by occupancy and season and time. You can call their Reservations number 520-742-6000 and ask for the military rate or you can go online at www.starwoodhotels.com or www.westinlapalomaresort.com and get the military rate for your next much needed relaxing stay at the Westin La Paloma Resort.

Tubac Golf Resort

1 Otero Road
Tubac, AZ 85646
520-398-2211
www.tubacgolfresort.com

Tubac Golf Resort offers a special rate for active duty military only, seven days a week. You must show a copy of military orders or proof of being active duty. Veterans and disable veterans can also get this special rate if they ask for it and there are rooms available. You must show a
valid military ID when you check-in.

Westgate Painted Mountain Resort

6302 East McKellips Road
Mesa, AZ 85215
480-654-3611
Rental Reservations: 1-888-433-3707
www.westgatedestinations.com

Westgate Painted Mountain Resort offers a 10% military discount for active duty and retired military and is based on availability. You have to call or you can book online. You need to show a valid military ID card when you check-in.

Westin Kierland Resort and Spa

6902 East Greenway Parkway
Scottsdale, AZ 85254
480-264-1000
www.kierlandresort.com

Westin Kierland Resort and Spa offers a government rate for government employees and active duty military. This rate is based on availability and demand. You must show a valid military ID and proof of being on active duty when you check-in.

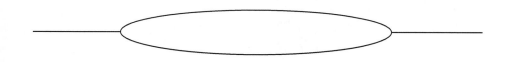

Westward Look Resort

245 East Ina Road
Tucson, AZ 85704
520-297-1151
www.wyndham.com/hotels/arizona/tucson/
westward-look-wyndham-grand-resort-and-spa
www.westwardlook.com

The Resort offers a military rate that varies by occupancy and season. You can call their reservations number or go online at one of the websites listed above and get the special rate as well.

The White Stallion Ranch

9251 West Twin Peaks Road
Tucson, AZ 85743
520-297-0252
www.wsranch.com

The White Stallion Ranch offers a 50% discount for active duty military during non-peak season and 20% discount during peak season. There is also a discount of 20% for retired military year-round. You can call in your reservation or you can book one online. You must show proof of being on active duty to get the discount and you must show a valid military ID when you check-in. Giddy up!!

Wyndham Green Valley Canoa Ranch Resort

5775 South Camino Del Sol
Green Valley, AZ 85622
520-382-0450
www.canoaranchgolfresort.com

Wyndham Canoa Ranch Resort offers a current government rate for military and veterans. You have to ask for this government rate. You can call in your reservation or you can book one online. You must show a valid military ID when you check-in.

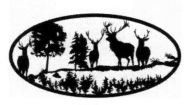

134

Arizona Bed and Breakfast Inns

Each year, the B&B industry celebrates the sacrifices offered by our courageous veterans by offering free rooms on or around Veteran's Day. In order to accommodate all those deserving free stays, innkeepers may offer "first-timers" to the program priority for stays. While others offer discounted rates all year-round. There are Bed and Breakfast Inns all over Arizona, from the cool pine mountainous beauty of Northern Arizona, the Red Rock country of Sedona, the lushness of Oak Canyon, the majestic beauty of Flagstaff, the Colorado communities of Lake Havasu and Parker, Scottsdale, Phoenix, Tucson, the beautiful White Tank Mountains and the popular Grand Canyon.

There's a tranquil Bed and Breakfast Inn just waiting for you. Just visit the website listed by each one to see what they have to offer you.

Adobe Rose Inn
940 North Olsen Avenue
Tucson, AZ 85719
520-318-4644
1-800-328-4122 Toll Free
www.adoberoseinn.com

Free room to active duty military or veterans to say thank you for your service during Veterans Day weekend. At least one room is available. First come, first served. Please contact the innkeeper@aroseinn.com for more information and to book your reservation.

Alma de Sedona Inn
50 Hozoni Drive
Sedona, AZ 86336
928-282-2734
www.almadesedona.com

One free night is available to military personnel with valid ID card during Veterans Day weekend. Full breakfast in the morning. Extend your stay before or after with additional nights at our discounted rates! Thanks for your service!

A Sunset Chateau

665 Sunset Drive
Sedona, AZ 86336
928-282-2644
www.asunsetchateau.com

A Sunset Chateau offers a 10% discount for military and veterans. You can call in your reservation or book one online. You must show a valid military ID when you check-in.

Boots and Saddles Bed and Breakfast

2900 Hopi Drive
Sedona, AZ 86336
928-282-1944
www.oldwestbb.com

Boots and Saddles offers $15 a night discount for active military only. You can call in your reservation or book one online. When you do book online, just let them know that you are active duty military and they will send you a corrected confirmation showing the discount. You must show documentation that you are on active duty and you must show a valid military ID when you check-in.

Briar Patch Inn

3190 North State Route 89A
Sedona, AZ 86336
928-282-2342
1-888-809-3030
www.briarpatchinn.com

The Briar Patch Inn offers a 10% military discount, 7 days a week. You can call in a reservation or book one online. When you book online, you can say that you are military in "guest notes". And they will honor the discount at check-in. You must show a valid military ID card at check-in.

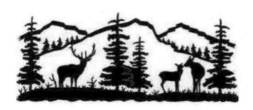

Canyon Colors Bed and Breakfast

225 South Navajo
Page, AZ 86040
928-645-5979
www.canyoncolorsbandb.com

Canyon Colors Bed and Breakfast offers a 10% discount for military and for veterans. You must show a valid military ID when you check-in.

Canyon Villa Bed and Breakfast Inn of Sedona

40 Canyon Circle Drive
Sedona, AZ 86351
928-284-1226
www.canyonvilla.com

Canyon Villa Bed and Breakfast Inn of Sedona offers a 10% discount to the U.S. Military, Active and Veterans and First Responders, Police Officers, Firemen, and EMS Crews. A 10% discounted rate applies to your entire reservation even if you only stay 1 night and applies to **ALL** guestrooms. This cannot be combined with any other room discount promotions and you must book directly with Canyon Villas. Documentation required upon arrival.

Casa Tierra Adobe Bed and Breakfast Inn

11155 West Calle Pima
Tucson, AZ 85743
520-578-3058
www.casatierratucson.com

Casa Tierra Adobe Bed & Breakfast Inn offers a free night to Veterans on and around Veterans Day. Must book directly at the number listed above or by booking a reservation online at the website listed above. Have a great stay and a better time!

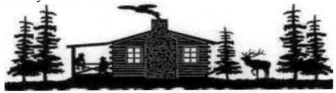

Catalina Park Inn Bed and Breakfast

309 East 1st Street
Tucson, AZ 85705
520-792-4541
www.catalinaparkinn.com

Catalina Park Inn Bed and Breakfast offers $10 off the normal going rate for active duty military *ONLY*. You must show current military orders or other proof of being on active duty.

You can call in your reservation or you can book it online. You must show a valid military ID when you check-in.

Cozy Cactus Bed and Breakfast

80 Canyon Circle Drive
Sedona, AZ 86351
928-284-0082
www.cozycactus.com

Cozy Cactus has a military discount that's 'not official'. Discount is based on their current room rate at the time and is based on season and the length of your stay. You can call in your reservation or book one online. You must show a valid military ID when you check-in.

Creekside Inn

99 Copper Cliffs Drive
Sedona, AZ 86336
928-282-4992
www.creekside.net

Creekside Inn Bed and Breakfast offers a 10% discount for active duty only. You must go to www.creekside.net and make a reservation and then you will have the opportunity to request the discount in guest notes. You must show a valid military ID card when you check-in.

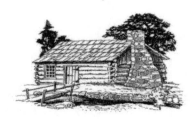

Desert Trails Bed & Breakfast

12851 East Speedway Blvd.
Tucson, AZ 85748
520-885-7295
1-877-758-3284 Toll Free
www.deserttrails.com

Desert Trails offers a discount for Active Duty ONLY. Discount varies by season and availability. You can call in your reservation or you can book one online. You must show a valid military ID card when you check-in.

Heritage Inn Bed and Breakfast

161 North Main Street
Snowflake, AZ 85937
928-536-3322
www.heritage-inn.net

Heritage Inn Bed and breakfast offers a 10% military discount. You will need to tell them you are military and ask for the discount. You must show a valid military ID when you check-in.

Indian Hill Bed and Breakfast

2955 North Tomahawk Trail
Tucson, AZ 85749
520-760-4200
www.indianhillbb.com

Indian Hill Bed and Breakfast offers a military discount for active duty military ONLY. You can call in your reservation or you can book one online. You have to ask for the discount and must show proof of being on active duty and you must show a valid military ID when you check-in.

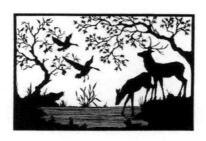

Inn at Civano

10448 East Seven Generations Way
Tucson, AZ 85747-5809
520-296-5428
www.innatciavano.com

The Inn at Civano offers one night free during Veterans Day weekend, (Sunday or Monday), double occupancy. Additional nights are only $80.00 a night with this promotion. Includes all fees and full breakfast for two. And there is a military and veterans discount that varies by season and availability. There is a code: vet1 (that is the word vet and the number one) for online reservations.

Maricopa Manor Bed and Breakfast Inn

15 West Pasadena Avenue
Phoenix, AZ 85013
602-264-9200
1-800-292-6403 Toll Free
www.maricopamanor.com

Maricopa Manor offers a 10% discount for military and veterans. You can call in your reservation or you can book one online. You must show a valid military ID when you check-in.

Prescott Pines Inn

901 White Spar Road
Prescott, AZ 86303
928-445-7270
www.prescottpinesinn.com

Prescott Pines Inn offers the first 5 premium rooms go to Veterans during the Veterans Day timeframe. You must go to the Bed and Breakfasts for Veterans website, www.bandbsforvets.org to register ***Thank you for your service!***

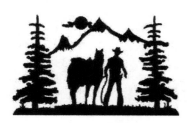

Red Garter Inn

137 West Railroad Avenue
Williams, AZ 86046
928-635-1484
1-800-328-1484 Toll Free
www.redgarter.com

The Red Garter Bed and Breakfast Inn offers a 10% discount for military and veterans. Reservations must be made through their website, www.redgarter.com. In the notes 'section' you can type in that you are military, or a veteran and they will take care of the discount for you. They also offer one room free available during the Veteran's Day timeframe so call early to see if it is still available. You must show a valid military ID when you check-in.

Sam Hughes Inn Bed and Breakfast

2020 East 7th Street
Tucson, AZ 85719
520-861-2191
www.samhughesinn.com

Sam Hughes Inn Bed and Breakfast offers the current government rate for recently served military and veterans (back to Desert Storm only). It is based on season and availability. You must provide proof that you had been recently serving in the military and you must show a valid military ID when you check-in.

Starlight Pines Bed and Breakfast

3380 East Lockett Road
Flagstaff, AZ 86004
928-527-1912
1-800-752-1912 Toll Free
www.starlightpinesbb.com

The Starlight Pines Bed and Breakfast offers a 10% discount for a 1-night stay and 15% discount on a two or more-night stay for military and veterans. You can call in your reservation or you can book one online. You must show a valid military ID when you check-in.

The Lodge of Sedona

125 Kallof Plave
Sedona, AZ 86336
928-204-1942
www.lodgeatsedona.com

One free night is available to military personnel with valid ID card during Veterans Day weekend. Full breakfast in the morning. Extend your stay before or after with additional nights at our discounted seasonal rates! Thanks for your service!

The Inns at El Rancho Merlita

1924 North Corte El Rancho Merlita
Tucson, AZ 85715
520-495-0071
www.ranchomerlita.com

The Inns at El Rancho Merlita offers a discount of $10 off the regular going room rate for active duty military and retired military. You must mention that you read about the discount in this book and they will honor the discount all year round. You can call in your reservation or you can book one online. You must show a valid military ID when you check-in.

Arizona Casinos

This is a list of Arizona Casinos that offer a Military / Veterans Appreciation Program of some sort. Special deals, free bonus play, discounts, it's all done to show our military and veterans that they are not forgotten. So, go have some fun!

Bucky's Casino

1500 East State Route 69
Prescott, AZ 86301
928-776-5695
1-800-756-8744-- Toll Free / www.buckyscasino.com

Bucky's Casino offers $10 in play and double points every Monday to veterans. You must sign up for the Gold Rush Club Program Veterans Card. You must show proof of being a veteran.

Casino Del Sol

1-800-SOL-STAY
    (765-7829)
www.casinoofthesun.com

The hotel at the casino usually offers a 10% military discount off of the going rate and when available. You can call the casino for more details. You must show a valid military ID card when you check-in.

Casino of the Sun

7406 South De Oeste Cami
Tucson, AZ 85746
520-883-1700
www.casinodelsol.com

Casino of the Sun offers a military discount at their café/snack bar of 10% to military and veterans. You must show a valid military ID card.

Desert Diamond Casino

7350 South Nogales Highway
Tucson, AZ 85756
520-214-7777
www.ddcaz.com

All Desert Diamond Casinos offer a Tribute Card for all Active & Retired Military. This card entitles you to $10 in free play twice a month, 12 complimentary hotel stays a year, free concert tickets to select shows and so much more. You have to sign up at any of their 3 current locations. Must provide either a valid military ID, or a CAC Card, or a DD Form 2 Card, or a DD Form 214 at their Rewards Center located at all of their casinos.

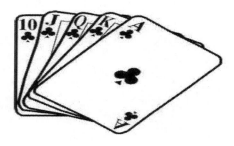

Desert Diamond Casino

Highway 86, Milepost 55
Ajo, AZ 85321
520-294-7777
www.ddcaz.com/why

All Desert Diamond Casinos offer a Tribute Card for all Active &
Retired Military. This card entitles you to $10 in free play twice a
month, 12 complimentary hotel stays a year, free concert tickets to
select shows and so much more. You have to sign up at any of their
3 current locations.

Must provide either a valid military ID, or a CAC Card, or a DD Form
2 Card, or a DD Form 214 at their Rewards Center located at all of
their casinos.

Desert Diamond Hotel – Casino

1100 West Pima Mine Road
Sahaurita, AZ 85629
520-294-7777
1-866-DDC-WINS
       (332-9467)
www.ddcaz.com/sahaurita

All Desert Diamond Casinos offer a Tribute Card for all Active &
Retired Military. This card entitles you to $10 in free play twice a
month, 12 complimentary hotel stays a year, free concert tickets to
select shows and so much more.

You have to sign up at any of their three current locations. Must
provide either a valid military ID, or a CAC Card, or a DD Form 2
Card, or a DD Form 214 at their Rewards Center located at all of
their casinos.

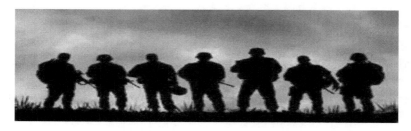

Gila River Casino - Lone Butte

1200 South 56th Street
Chandler, AZ 85246
1-800-946-4452
www.wingilariver.com/lonebutte

MILITARY MONDAYS - Every Monday from 7 am to 3 pm military Players Club Members can swipe their Players Club Card and win up to $100 Free Bonus Play plus receive 15% off select food and Gift Shop purchases.

You must present a valid Players Club Card, a valid military ID and any proof of Military service to the Lone Butte Players Club. Military requirements vary for age verification, reportable transactions, Players Club memberships and sale of tobacco and alcohol products. See Players Club for more details.

You have to show proof of military service at Players Club to participate. You have to sign up to be a Players Club Member.

Gila River Casino - Vee Quiva

6443 North Kamatka Lane
Laverne, AZ 85339
1-800-946-4452
www.wingilariver.com/vee-quiva

SWIPES FOR SOLDIERS - Every Wednesday from 7 am to 3 pm active duty and retired military can swipe their Players Club card for a chance to win up to $100 Free Bonus Play and receive a 15% discount on select food, beverage or retail items. You have to show proof of military service at Players Club to participate. You have to sign up to be a Players Club Member.

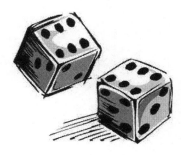

Gila River Casino – Wild Horse Pass Hotel & Casino

5040 Wildhorse Pass Blvd.
Chandler, AZ 85226
1-800-946-4452
www.wingilariver.com/wild-horse-pass

WARRIOR WEDNESDAYS -- Every Wednesday from 7 am to 3 pm active duty and retired military Players Club Card members can swipe their Players Club card for a chance instantly win! You could win up to $100 in Free Bonus Play instantly. Visit Players Club for your 20% off food voucher, good at any restaurant at Wild Horse Pass Hotel & Casino, except Shula's Steakhouse.

You have to show proof of military service at Players Club to participate. And you have to sign up to be a Players Club Member.

Yavapai Casino

1505 East State Route 69
Prescott, AZ 86301
928-445-9767
1-800-756-8744—Toll Free
www.buckyscasino.com

Yavapai Casino offers $10 free-play and double-points every Monday to veterans. You must sign up for the Gold Rush Club Program Veterans Card. You must show proof of being a veteran.

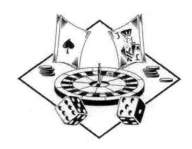

This is a list of Arizona Casinos that do not offer a Military /Veterans Appreciation Program, but do offer specials, free bonus play, discounts and other deals for our veterans throughout the year.

Bluewater Resort and Casino
11300 Resort Drive
Parker, AZ 85344
928-669-7777
www.bluewatercasino.com

Casino Arizona
524 North 92nd Street
Scottsdale, AZ 85256
480-850-7777
www.casinoarizona.com

Cliff Castle Casino
555 W. Middle Verde Rd.
Camp Verde, AZ 86322
928-567-6611
www.cliffcastlecasinohotel.com

Hon-Dah Resort Casino
777 North Highway 260
Pinetop, AZ 85935
1-800-929-8744
www.hon-dah.com

Talking Stick Casino
9800 E. Indian Bend Rd.
Scottsdale, AZ 85256
480-850-7777
www.talkingstick resort.com

Cocopah Casino and Bingo
15318 South Avenue B
Somerton, AZ 85350
928-217-8066
1-800-23-SLOTS (7-5687)
www.cocopahresort.com

Fort McDowell Casino
10424 North Fort McDowell Road
Fort McDowell, AZ 85264
602-843-3678
www.fortmcdowellcasino.com

Spirit Mountain Casino
8555 South Highway
Mohave Valley, AZ 86440
928-346-2000

Mazatzal Casino
Highway 89, MP #251
Payson, AZ 85547
928-474-6044
1-800-777-PLAY (7529)
www.mazatzal-casino.com

Paradise Casino
450 Quechan Drive
Yuma, AZ 85364
760-572-7777
1-800-777-4946
www.paradise-casinos.com

Veterans Advantage

Travel & Entertainment Discounts for Veterans, Military & Families

www.veteransadvantage.com

Veterans Advantage salutes your military service with a full range of discounts from travel like airline, train, bus, cruise and rental car discounts -- plus travel booking services. From major cruise line discounts, Disney tickets, sports ticket discounts, vacation rentals, hotel reservations, movie ticket discounts, National Parks, Zoos and Aquariums, PGA TOUR and Champions Tour Golf tickets and many, many more.

The Veterans Advantage Card Benefits Program has been created to provide greater recognition, respect, and rewards for all who have served in the U.S. Military, including Veterans, Active Duty Military, National Guard and Reserves, and their family members. You qualify from any branch of service and rank, period of service, or length of service.

As soon as you enroll, you will receive your Veterans Advantage Card, personalized with your name and branch of service, and be eligible for special offers from top corporations who wish to honor and thank you for your service. We make all efforts to let you know your benefits exist, too - online, direct to your mailbox, and through our toll-free member support hotline.

At Veterans Advantage, we believe when one family member serves, the whole family serves. Family members who are "next of kin" may enroll as the spouse, mother, father, daughter or son of the Veteran or Serviceperson and are eligible for special benefits too.

 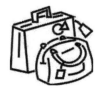

Cruise Line Discounts

From time to time, one or more cruise lines will offer special discounts or ship-board credits on select sailings for Vacations to Go customers who are members of the military. In some cases, Active, reserve, and retired members of the U.S. Military and the Canadian Forces may be eligible. Veterans may also be eligible with some cruise lines offering special discounts to veterans with an Honorable Discharge who have served in an active war zone for any length of time or outside a war zone for at least two years. Spouses of actively deployed or deceased military personnel may also be eligible. In select cases, U.S. Armed Forces Personnel in the following branches may be eligible: Army Corps of Engineers, Central Intelligence Agency, Federal Bureau of Investigation, National Security Agency (excluding Homeland Security), Secret Service, Naval Criminal Investigation Service (NCIS), NASA Kennedy Space Center, NASA Johnson Space Center, Department of Health and Human Services, and Cadets who are currently enrolled in a military academy with a scheduled entry date into the military. Military personnel must present proper documentation at the time of booking to qualify for the special rates.

CARNIVAL CRUISE LINES

Carnival Cruise Lines offers military discounts on select sailings to Active personnel currently serving in the United States Military, Air Force, Army, Coast Guard, Department of Health and Human Services, National Guard, Navy, Marines, and Reserves, as well as Cadets that are currently enrolled in a military academy with a scheduled entry date into one of these divisions. Retired personnel from any of these divisions are also eligible. "Retired" is defined as A) enlisted personnel or officers with a minimum of 20 years of service, B) medically retired, or C) 100 % disabled. Veterans with an honorable discharge serving a minimum of two years, or who served in an active war zone, in any of the United States service divisions listed above are also eligible. In addition, Active, reserve and retired Canadian National Defense personnel are also eligible for Carnival's military discounts. Finally, spouses of actively deployed or deceased military personnel are eligible to book one stateroom and others in the same stateroom will also be allowed to cruise at the military rate.

Qualifying guests must submit a photocopy of enlistment papers, LES Leave and Earning Statement), with the social security number blacked out, or discharge papers, (Form DD214 or DD256) and a passport or driver's license via fax to Carnival and Vacations to Go at the time of booking. Carnival will charge guests the standard market rate if they do not receive proper documentation within 48 hours of booking. www.carnival.com Phone: 1-800-764-7419.

CELEBRITY CRUISE LINES

Celebrity Cruise Lines offers military discounts on select sailings for Active or reserve personnel currently serving in the United States Army, Air Force, Navy, Marines, Coast Guard, and National Guard and the Canadian Forces, and retired personnel from any of these divisions. "Retired" is defined as A) enlisted personnel or officers with a minimum of 20 years of service, B) medically retired, or C) 100 % disabled. Veterans with an honorable discharge serving a minimum of two years, or 6 months in an active war zone, in any of the United States service divisions listed above are also eligible.

Finally, spouses of actively deployed or deceased military personnel are eligible to book one stateroom and others in the same stateroom will also be allowed to cruise at the military rate. Qualifying guests must submit a photocopy of proper military ID and a passport or driver's license at the time of booking. www.celebritycruises.com Phone: 1-800-647-2251.

COSTA CRUISE LINES

Costa Cruise Lines offers military discounts on select sailings for Active or reserve personnel currently serving in the United States Army, Army Corps of Engineers, Air Force, Navy, Naval Criminal Investigation Service (NCIS), Marines, Coast Guard, National Guard, the Canadian Forces, and retired personnel from any of these divisions. "Retired" is defined as A) enlisted personnel or officers with a minimum of 20 years of service, B) medically retired, or C) 100 % disabled. Veterans with an honorable discharge serving a minimum of two years, or who served in an active war zone, in any of the United States service divisions listed above are also eligible.

Finally, spouses of actively deployed or deceased military personnel are eligible to book one stateroom and others in the same stateroom will also be allowed to cruise at the military rate. Qualifying guests must submit a photocopy of proper military ID and a passport or driver's license at the time of booking. www.costacruise.com Phone: 1-800-GO COSTA.

DISNEY CRUISE LINES

Disney Cruise Lines offers military discounts on select sailings for Active or reserve personnel currently serving in the United States Army, Air Force, Navy, Marines, Coast Guard, National Guard, or Reserves and to the United States Department of Defense personnel and retired personnel from any of these divisions. "Retired" is defined as A) enlisted personnel or officers with a minimum of 20 years of service, B) medically retired, or C) 100 % disabled. Veterans with an honorable discharge who are 100 % permanently disabled are eligible. A valid military ID card with the code of DAVPRM printed on the front is required for veterans. Qualifying guests must submit a photocopy of proper military ID and a passport or driver's license at the time of booking. www.disneycruise.com Phone: 1-800-951-3532.

HOLLAND AMERICA

For more than 140 years, Holland America has been a recognized leader in cruising, taking our guests to exotic destinations around the world. If you are looking for some of the most spacious and comfortable ships at sea, award-winning service, five-star dining, extensive activities and enrichment programs and compelling worldwide itineraries, you've come to the right place.

We are committed to our mission: through excellence, we create once-in-a-lifetime experiences, every time. Holland America offers military discounts on select sailings for Active personnel currently serving in the Canadian Forces, United States Army, Air Force, Navy, Marines, Coast Guard, National Guard, or Merchant Marines. Qualifying guests must submit a photocopy of proper military ID and a passport or driver's license at the time of booking. www.hollandamerica.com Phone: 1-877-932-4259.

MSC CRUISES

MCS Cruises offers military discounts on select sailings for Active or reserve personnel currently serving in the United States Army, Air Force, Navy, Marines, Coast Guard, National Guard and the Canadian Forces as well as U.S. Armed Forces Personnel in the following branches: Central Intelligence Agency, Federal Bureau of Investigation, National Security Agency (excluding Homeland Security), Secret Service, Naval Criminal Investigation Service (NCIS), NASA Kennedy Space Center, NASA Johnson Space Center, Department of Health and Human Services, and Cadets who are currently enrolled in a military academy with a scheduled entry date into the military. Retired personnel from any of these divisions are also eligible. "Retired" is defined as A) enlisted personnel or officers with a minimum of 20 years of service, B) medically retired, or C) 100 % disabled. Veterans with an honorable discharge serving a minimum of two years, or who served in an active war zone, in any of the United States service divisions listed above are also eligible. Finally, spouses of actively deployed or deceased military personnel are eligible to book one stateroom at the military rate.

The spouse of the military member must be booked in the stateroom and others in the same stateroom will also be allowed to cruise at the military rate. Qualifying guests must submit a photocopy of proper military ID and a passport or driver's license at the time of booking. www.msccruises.com Phone: 1-877-665-4655.

NORWEGIAN CRUISE LINE

Norwegian Cruise Lines offers military discounts on select sailings for Active or reserve personnel currently serving in the United States Army, Army Corps of Engineers, Air Force, Navy, Marines, Coast Guard, National Guard and the Canadian Forces, and Naval Criminal Investigation Service (NCIS), and retired personnel from any of these divisions are also eligible. "Retired" is defined as A) enlisted personnel or officers with a minimum of 20 years of service, B) medically retired, or C) 100 % disabled.

Veterans with an honorable discharge serving a minimum of two years, in an active war zone, in any of the United States service divisions listed above are also eligible. Finally, spouses of actively deployed or deceased military personnel are eligible to book one stateroom at the military rate. The spouse of the military member must be booked in the stateroom and others in the same stateroom will also be allowed to cruise at the military rate. Qualifying guests must submit a photocopy of proper military ID and a passport or driver's license at the time of booking. www.NCL.com Phone: 1-866-234-7350.

PRINCESS CRUISE LINES

Princess Cruise Lines offers shipboard credits on select sailings for Active or reserve personnel currently serving in the United States Army, Air Force, Navy, Marines, Coast Guard, National Guard and the Canadian Forces, and Reserves as well as retired personnel from any of these divisions are also eligible. "Retired" is defined as A) enlisted personnel or officers with a minimum of 20 years of service, B) medically retired, or C)100 % disabled. Veterans with an honorable discharge serving a minimum of two years, or 6 months in an active war zone, in any of the United States service divisions listed above are also eligible. Qualifying guests must submit a photocopy of proper military ID and a passport or driver's license at the time of booking. Shipboard credits are valued at $50 per person on all cruises of 6-nights or less, $100 per person on cruises of 7 to 13 nights, and $250 per person on cruises of 14 nights or longer, with a maximum of two onboard credits per stateroom.

This promotion is combinable with other shipboard credit offers listed on individual sailings, but it may not be combinable with all fares. www.princess.com Phone: 1-855-632-6259 or 1-800-774-6237.

PULLMANTUR CRUISES

Pullmantur Cruises offers military discounts on select sailings for Active or reserve personnel currently serving in the United States Army, Air Force, Navy, Marines, Coast Guard, National Guard and the Canadian Forces as well as U.S. Armed Forces Personnel in the following branches: Central Intelligence Agency, Federal Bureau of Investigation, National Security Agency (excluding Homeland Security), Secret Service, Naval Criminal Investigation Service (NCIS), NASA

153

Kennedy Space Center, NASA Johnson Space Center, Department of Health and Human Services, and Cadets who are currently enrolled in a military academy with a scheduled entry date into the military. Retired personnel from any of these divisions are also eligible. "Retired" is defined as A) enlisted personnel or officers with a minimum of 20 years of service, B) medically retired, or C) 100 % disabled. Veterans with an honorable discharge serving a minimum of two years, or who served in an active war zone, in any of the United States service divisions listed above are also eligible as are all Veterans Advantage members. Finally, spouses of actively deployed or deceased military personnel are eligible to book one stateroom at the military rate. The spouse of the military member must be booked in the stateroom and others in the same stateroom will also be allowed to cruise at the military rate. Qualifying guests must submit a photocopy of proper military ID and a passport or driver's license at the time of booking. www.pullmanturcruiseline.com Phone: 1-888-381-4656.

ROYAL CARIBBEAN

Royal Caribbean offers military discounts on select sailings for Active or reserve personnel currently serving in the United States Army, Air Force, Navy, Marines, Coast Guard, National Guard, the Canadian Forces, and retired personnel from any of these divisions. "Retired" is defined as A) enlisted personnel or officers with a minimum of 20 years of service, B) medically retired, or C) 100 % disabled. Veterans with an honorable discharge serving a minimum of two years, or 6-months in an active war zone, in any of the United States service divisions listed above are also eligible. Finally, spouses of actively deployed or deceased military personnel are eligible to book one stateroom. The spouse of the military member must be booked in the stateroom and others in the same stateroom will also be allowed to cruise at the military rate.

Qualifying guests must submit a photocopy of proper military ID and a passport or driver's license at the time of booking. www.royalcarribbean.com Phone: 1-866-562-7625.

VOYAGES OF DISCOVERY

Voyages of Discovery offers military discounts on select sailings for Active or reserve personnel currently serving in the United States Army, Air Force, Navy, Marines, Coast Guard, National Guard and the Canadian Forces as well as U.S. Armed Forces Personnel in the following branches: Central Intelligence Agency, Federal Bureau of Investigation, National Security Agency (excluding Homeland Security), Secret Service, Naval Criminal Investigation Service (NCIS), NASA Kennedy Space Center, NASA Johnson Space Center, Department of Health and Human Services, and Cadets who are currently enrolled in a military academy with a scheduled entry date into the military. Retired personnel from any of these divisions are also eligible. "Retired" is defined as A) enlisted personnel or officers with a minimum of 20 years of service, B) medically retired, or C) 100 % disabled. Veterans with an honorable discharge serving a minimum of two years, or who served in an active war zone, in any of the United States service divisions listed above are also eligible as are all Veterans Advantage members. Finally, spouses of actively deployed or deceased military personnel are eligible to book one stateroom at the military rate. The spouse of the military member must be booked in the stateroom and others in the same stateroom will also be allowed to cruise at the military rate. Qualifying guests must submit a photocopy of proper military ID and a passport or driver's license at the time of booking.
www.us.voyagesofdiscovery.com. Phone; 1-866-623-2689.

VOYAGES OF ANTIQUITIES

Voyages of Antiquities offers military discounts on select sailings for Active or reserve personnel currently serving in the United States Army, Air Force, Navy, Marines, Coast Guard, National Guard and the Canadian Forces as well as U.S. Armed Forces Personnel in the following branches: Central Intelligence Agency, Federal Bureau of Investigation, National Security Agency (excluding Homeland Security), Secret Service, Naval Criminal Investigation Service (NCIS), NASA Kennedy Space Center, NASA Johnson Space Center, Department of Health and Human Services, and Cadets who are currently enrolled in a military academy with a scheduled entry date into the military. Retired personnel from any of these divisions are also eligible.

"Retired" is defined as A) enlisted personnel or officers with a minimum of 20 years of service, B) medically retired, or C) 100 % disabled. Veterans with an honorable discharge serving a minimum of two years, or who served in an active war zone, in any of the United States service divisions listed above are also eligible as are all Veterans Advantage members. Finally, spouses of actively deployed or deceased military personnel are eligible to book one stateroom at the military rate.

The spouse of the military member must be booked in the stateroom and others in the same stateroom will also be allowed to cruise at the military rate. Qualifying guests must submit a photocopy of proper military ID and a passport or driver's license at the time of booking. www.voyagesofantiquities.com Phone: 1-877-398-1460.

AMERICAN CRUISE LINES

American Cruise Lines offers world-class, small ship cruises along the inland waterways and rivers of the United States. From the Mississippi River to the New England and Alaska, our modern fleet of ships and paddle wheelers are the perfect way to see America.

Highly personalized service and a relaxed atmosphere prevails onboard all our modern fleet of ships. Our accommodating, all-American crew welcomes you with an unequaled level of attention. Each evening before dinner, enjoy complimentary cocktails and hors oeuvres, as you mingle with other passengers to exchange the adventures of the day. Set your own pace on your vacation and relish in the casual comfort and exceptional care that is the hallmark of the cruising with American Cruise Lines.

Enjoy superb refinement on the newest ships built in the USA. Relax in finely appointed staterooms that are among the largest in the world while our attentive staff creates a personalized cruise experience where your every desire is met with care and precision.

2015 cruise itineraries include Mississippi River cruises, Pacific Northwest cruises, New England, Mid-Atlantic and Southwest US cruises from 7 to 14 nights. www.americancruiselines.com Phone: 1-800-460-4518 or 1-800-814-6880.

QUARK EXPEDITIONS

Quark Expeditions is specialized in expedition cruising to the Artic and Antarctica, in ships with ice-strengthened hulls or in icebreakers. Polar travelers will enjoy unparalleled technical expertise, leadership and passion for expedition trips to the Artic and Antarctica.

We have the largest and most diverse fleet of adventure ships in the Antarctica and Artic. Travelers choose from more departures and a greater variety of itineraries that is available anywhere else. Within the fleet is the only nuclear-powered icebreaker – 50 Years of Victory – sailing to the North Pole. Every ship is equipped with Zodiacs-inflatable landing craft-for shore transfers and ocean-level cruising. Our Polar Adventure Ships are platforms for optional sea-kayaking, camping, mountaineering and cross-country skiing.

Their small size enables them to sail channels and bays through which our icebreakers cannot sail. The ability to get close to landscapes and wildlife make these vessels extraordinary base camps for photographers.

None of our vessels carries more than 128 travelers from around the world – Europe, Asia, Oceania, North America and Africa. They all share a preference for travel to remote wilderness areas accompanied by Expedition Team Member's eager to share their knowledge and love for the Artic and Antarctica. www.quarkexpeditions.com Phone: 1-888-978-9756 or 1-802-490-7806 (outside North America).

REGENT SEVEN SEAS CRUISES

Regent Seven Seas Cruises fleet includes sister all-suite, all-balcony, 700-guest ships Seven Seas Voyager and Seven Seas Mariner, and the all-suite, 90% balcony Seven Seas navigator. Regent Seven Seas Cruises, with headquarters in Miami, is owned by Prestige Cruise Holdings, the market leader in the Upper Premium and Luxury segments of the cruise industry with over 6,400 berths between the Regent Seven Seas Cruises and Oceania Cruises brands. www.rssc.com/RegentSevenSeasCruises Phone: 1-877-505-5370.

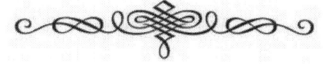

SEABOURN CRUISES

Seabourn Cruises are passionate about travel. We believe that traveling for pleasure has a redemptive power that enriches people's lives. And we believe that people should travel well. Cruising on a Seabourn ship is unlike any other form of travel. The experience is luxurious, yet relaxed-elegant, yet casual-sumptuous, yet understated. Our intimate ships visit the most desirable destinations worldwide, sailing to the heart of landmark cities, as well as to hidden gems where larger vessels cannot follow.

Our ships attract interesting people, who seek to share experiences beyond the expected in places beyond the ordinary. Our acclaimed staff offers a unique style of heartfelt hospitality that is sincere, thoughtful and personal. www.seabourn.com Phone: 1-877-293-7153.

UNIWORLD RIVER CRUISES

Uniworld River Cruises offers the highest level of comfort, quality, and service in river cruising with an unparalleled variety of vacation choices. For nearly 40 years, Uniworld River Cruises has taken guests to the world's greatest destinations – Asia, Europe, Egypt, and Russia. You'll cherish the ultimate first-class European boutique, hotel-style cruise experience when sailing with Uniworld River Cruises. take you to a plethora of destinations unreachable by large cruise ships. Geared toward the experienced traveler, Uniworld River Cruises take guests beyond the typical tourist sites.

You will find knowledgeable, English-speaking guides and staff on every tour, plus something else – American style amenities, accommodations, and cuisine. Uniworld River Cruises ships are also famous for their sociable, friendly atmospheres, so be prepared to meet some new friends and create lifetime memories.

Uniworld River Cruises offers a unique river cruise vacation experience for travelers and will www.uniworldcruises.com Phone: 1-888-234-8369.

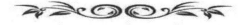

WINDSTAR LUXURY CRUISES

Windstar's small ship luxury cruises feel like your own private yacht – luxurious amenities, gourmet cuisine, exceptional service, and unique and exotic ports of call. With fewer than 300 guests, Windstar's yachts are small enough to reach places other ships cannot go, yet large enough to pamper and entertain you. Sail to the Greek Isles, Italy, Europe, the azure waters of the Caribbean, and the lush paradise of Tahiti. Windstar's yacht style cruises give you the ultimate luxury – freedom. www.windstarcruises.com Phone: 1-877-690-7036.

AZAMARA CLUB CRUISES

Azamara Club Cruises are always continuing their efforts to be the world's top up-market cruise line. As such, we are committed to providing you with unparalleled service; the finest dining at sea; a glorious spa and wellness experience. With our hallmark of longer stays, over nights and night touring, we not only take you to awe-inspiring destinations, but also give you more time to fall in love with them. www.azamaraclubcruises.com Phone: 1-877-999-9553.

PEARL SEAS CRUISES

Pearl Seas Cruises defines Luxury Adventure every day with an exceptional small-ship cruise experience that brings the world's most majestic cruise destinations, diverse cultures and stunning natural beauty to life. Join us aboard the n Pearl Mist for a backstage pass to the culture, customs and cuisine of the world's most majestic cruise destinations – many of which are not accessible by large ships. Enjoy a 7,10, 11 or 14-night cruise on the Great Lakes, St. Lawrence Seaway, West Indies, or Panama Canal.

Let Pearl Seas introduce you to the personalized service, fine dining, enriching onboard activities and guided shore excursions that are the hallmark of small-ship cruising with Pearl Seas. www.pearlseas.com Phone: 1-800-981-9146.

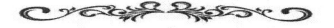

Space-Available Travel

Space-available travel is a service offered by the Department of Defense which provides unused seats on military flights to current and retired service members and their families looking to travel at little to no cost. However, families of reservists, including Gray Area Soldiers, are prevented from flying Space-A until the sponsor qualifies for retired pay and has a blue ID card.

Travelers should understand that the primary mission of the Air Mobility Command (AMC) is the movement of space required (duty) passengers and cargo on Department of Defense owned or controlled aircraft.

Although Space-A flights are free (commercial chartered flights charge a $15 - $30 fee), there are no guaranteed seats.

But if you're up for an adventure, and have a bit of patience, Space-A travel can be a ton of fun! Flight schedules for Space-A are released three days ahead of the planned departures and seat availability is listed as early as two to three hours before the flight. Passengers are also ranked in six categories by order of priority, depending on the importance of the travel, with emergency leave listed as 'Category 1' and Retired Soldiers listed as 'Category VI'. Passengers can register for a flight in five ways: in person, fax, email, internet or mail and the earlier the passenger is registered, the higher priority they have within their travel category.

There are several bases to travel out of. Here are just a few:

> Ramstein Air Base in Germany
> Travis Air Force Base in California
> Yokota Air Base in Japan
> Aviano Air Base in Italy
> Baltimore-Washington IAP in Maryland
> MacDill Air Force Base in Florida
> Lajes Air Base in Azores Portugal

Travelers can find more details about the Space-A Program at the following websites:

www.amc.af.mil/amctravel
www.facebook.com/notes/joint-base-pearl-harbor-hickam-amc-passenger-terminal/faqs-space-a-travel/362787953790620

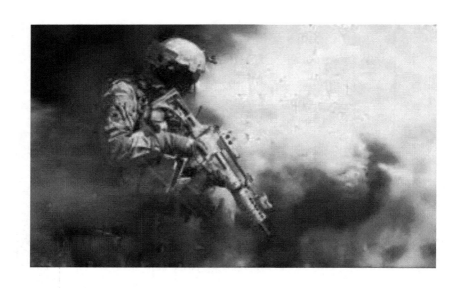

May no Soldier
go unloved

May no Soldier
walk alone

May no Soldier
be forgotten

May no Soldier
be left behind
when they return

Organizations that Assist Veterans in Need

"There is a time to take counsel of your fears, and there is a time to never listen to any fear. " – Gen. George S. Patton

Members of the military courageously volunteer to serve the United States. Their sacrifices include spending time away from their families and loved ones and getting sent to war zones. Unfortunately, military personnel can get injured while serving. Veteran organizations exist to help provide assistance to the veterans and their families. The services range from medical care to financial assistance.

FISHER HOUSE FOUNDATION

Injured military members and their families often have to travel for specializes medical care for the injured military member. The Fisher House Foundation provides houses – or 'comfort homes' for family members of patients on the grounds of VA Medical Centers and Military Installations at no cost. The houses provide up to 21 suites and can hold between 16 to 42 family members, which can be a great relief for families during a stressful time. A Fisher House contains a dining room, kitchen, laundry room and living room with a library and toys for the kids. The Foundation was established in 1990 when real estate developer Zachary Fisher and his wife Elizabeth M. Fisher gave more than $20 million for the construction of homes.

THE FISHER HOUSE FOUNDATION
111 Rockville Pike, Suite 420
Rockville, MD 20850-5168
1-888-294-8560
www.fisherhouse.org

INTREPID FALLEN HEROES FUND

The Fund has given more than $65 million to families of military members lost in service and for severely wounded veterans and military personnel, according to the organization. The Fund has provided grants to spouses and children of military members and built a $45 million, top-notch physical rehabilitation facility at Brooke Army Medical Center in San Antonio, Texas. On June 5, 2008, ground was broken on a 72,000-square foot facility adjacent to the Walter Reed National Military Medical Center on the Navy Campus at Bethesda, Maryland. It's intended to be a facility for the research, diagnosis and treatment of traumatic brain injury (TBI) and psychological health issues. The Fund began in 2000 as part of the Intrepid Museum Foundation. In 2003, it was established as an independent organization.

INTREPID FALLEN HEROES FUND
One Intrepid Square
West 46th Street and 12th Avenue
New York, New York 10036
www.fallenheroesfund.org/Home.aspx

THE ARMED SERVICES YMCA

The organization, which works with the Department of Defense, gives support services to military service personnel and their families. The focus is in helping junior-enlisted members with programs, including childcare, food services, hospital assistance and spouse support services. The Armed Services YMCA

ASYMCA has 16 branch locations, nine affiliated community YMCA's and six Department of Defense/Department of Homeland Security affiliates worldwide. The organization began during the Civil War when YMCA members provided volunteer relief to American Armed Forces.

THE ARMED FORCES YMCA
6359 Walker Lane, Suite 200
Alexandria, VA 22310
703-313-9600
www.asymca.org/Default.aspx

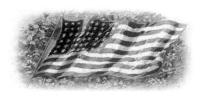

THE AMERICAN RED CROSS SOUTHERN ARIZONA CHAPTER

Service to the Armed Forces – Supporting Our Service Men and Women, Our Nation's Veterans and their families.

The American Red Cross Southern Arizona Chapter offers confidential services to all military personnel (Active duty, National Guard, Reserves, and Veterans) and their families by connecting them with resources through the Red Cross and our community partners, and in coordination with all branches of military service.

Military and Veteran families rely on the Red Cross to help them identify their needs and connect them to appropriate resources, ranging from responding to emergency needs for food, clothing, and shelter, referrals to financial and mental health counseling, respite care for caregivers, and other resources that meet their unique needs.

Our Programs

The American Red Cross, Southern Arizona Chapter Service to the Armed Forces Program supports Davis Monthan Air Force Base, Fort Huachuca, multiple regional military installations, the Veterans Administration Hospital and its satellite clinics.

Representing the 9th largest veteran population in the U.S., Southern Arizona is home to nearly 20,000 active duty military, and 100,000 veterans and their families.

Emergency Communication Services

The Red Cross is available around-the-clock to relay emergency messages to active duty service members, including notifications such as the death or serious illness of an immediate family member, as well as good news, like the birth of service member's child or grandchild.

Using advanced communications technologies to link service members and their families, our Emergency Communications Center quickly obtains and verifies the required information and sends emergency messages to service members, wherever in the world they happen to be.

Red Cross-verified information assists service members and their commanding officers in making decisions regarding emergency leave.

Information, Referral & Advocacy

They offer confidential services to all military personnel (active duty, National Guard, Reserves, and Veterans) and their families by connecting them with Red Cross and community resources, including:

- Benefits Information & Referral
- Employment & Education Support
- Counseling Support & Referrals
- Housing Assistance & Help with Utilities
- Transportation Assistance

Deployment Services

Before, during and after deployments, the Red Cross provides training, information and support for military members and their families. Being prepared to deal with challenges that may arise at home gives everyone peace of mind and helps the service member focus on the mission ahead.

- Get to Know Us Before You Need Us" briefings inform deploying troops and their families about Red Cross emergency services.
- Coping with Deployment:" classes help families build resiliency and respond to challenges during the deployment cycle.
- Reconnection Workshops assist those returning from deployment to adjust to family dynamics that may have changed while they were gone, work on communication skills, and develop coping mechanisms for stress or depression.

Emergency Financial Assistance

They offer a broad range of services to members of the military, veterans and their families, including access to emergency financial assistance. When an urgent personal or family crisis arises – call them. They may be able to help.

The Red Cross works with military aid societies from all service branches to provide financial assistance if needed.

Entitled Veterans Services

The Red Cross coordinates services such as navigating the benefits process, representing veterans and their families who seek compensation awards from the Department of Veterans Affairs (DVA) and helping wounded soldiers receive treatment at VA hospitals and clinics. Red Cross staff and volunteers also serve hospitalized veterans at VA medical centers with disaster assistance, health and safety education, and volunteer opportunities.

To find out more about Red Cross programs serving active military, National Guard, Reserves, Veterans and their families, call the Red Cross at 520-318-6740 or 1-800-341-6943, ext.#3678.

THE AMERICAN RED CROSS SOUTHERN ARIZONA CHAPTER
2916 East Broadway Blvd.
Tucson, AZ 85716
520-318-6740
1-800341-6943, ext. #3678
www.redcross.org/southernarizona

Arizona Military Family Relief Fund

The Arizona Military Relief Fund provides assistance for Active Duty Service Members, post 9/11 Veterans and their families. For families of currently deployed service members or service members injured or killed in action, financial assistance is available to assist with any unforeseen financial crises they might encounter.

For separated service members, financial assistance is available to assist with financial hardships caused by deployment to a combat zone. This includes, but is not limited to financial hardships caused by service-connected disabilities.

In order to qualify, the service member or veteran must clearly demonstrate the financial need was caused by their deployment and service.

Statutory Eligibility Requirements - Service Members and post 9/11 Veterans must meet all three eligibility requirements:

Deployment – Deployed to a designated combat zone after September 11, 2001

Arizona Residency (must meet one of these conditions)

> A). claimed Arizona as home of record when entering the Armed Forces, or
> B). deployed with the National Guard, or
> C). deployed from an Arizona military installation

Hardship – hardship occurred during deployment, or is caused, related or contributed to by deployment.

For more information and to apply, contact the Arizona Department of Veterans' Services or visit them at www.azdvs.gov

---

"The price of freedom is eternal vigilance." – Thomas Jefferson

U.S. Vets – Delivers Hope and Help to Veterans in Crisis.

HEADQUARTERS
800 West Sixth Street
Suite #1505
Los Angeles, CA 90017

Phone: 213-542-2600
Website: www.usvetsinc.org

U.S. Vets is a nonprofit 501(c) 3 corporation. With housing located in Barbers Point, HI and Waianae, HI; The District of Columbia; Houston, TX; Inglewood, CA; Las Vegas, NV; Long Beach, CA; Phoenix, AZ; Prescott, AZ; Riverside, CA

MISSION

"The successful transition of military veterans and their families through the provision of housing, counseling, career development and comprehensive support."

Imagine a veteran who comes home after a rigorous tour of duty, only to be faced with a new ordeal --- no job, no place in the community, the possibility of ending up homeless. For thousands of veterans who served their country honorably--- men and women alike---readjusting to civilian life is filled with uncertainties and obstacles. The battle isn't over. The battle to rebuild their lives has just begun.

- Since 1993, U.S. Vets has helped America's veterans make a successful transition back into their communities.
- Recognized as the largest national non-profit provider of comprehensive services to veterans.
- Operates programs at 11 sites in 5 states and the District of Columbia, with beds to accommodate more than 2,100 veterans every day.
- Collaborates with local area providers; Veterans Administration Medical Centers, and government agencies to help veterans get back on their feet.

PROGRAMS

VETERANS IN PROGRESS (VIP): A work re-entry program with a comprehensive approach that assists veterans to prepare for, obtain and maintain employment.

ADVANCE WOMEN'S PROGRAMS: A comprehensive program designed to meet the needs of female veterans, including a sexual trauma component.

VETERANS RE-ENTRY PROJECT (VRP): Provides a work re-entry program with a comprehensive approach that assists veterans to prepare for, obtain and maintain employment.

TRANSITIONAL AND AFFORDABLE PERMANENT HOUSING: Service enriched, sober housing for veterans with case management, meals, peer support, medical referrals and therapeutic groups.

CAREER CENTERS: State-of-the-art job search and training resources available to all veterans.

FATHERS PROGRAM: A program modeled after the VIP program and targets non-custodial fathers to help them become more emotionally and financially involved in their children's lives.

INCARCERATED VETERANS TRANSITITIONAL PROGRAM (IVTP): Provides on and off-site Case Management for veterans who are recently incarcerated or have been released within a six-month period. For this potentially hard to place population, additional services and skill sets are acquired through on-site case management and assistance for all veterans, as well as other community resources.

Each year:

- 3,000 veterans receive housing and comprehensive support services
- 1,100 veterans return to full-time employment.
- 250 disabled and senior veterans receive permanent housing.
- 700,000 meals are served at our sites throughout the U.S.

Cloudbreak Communities
414 South Marengo Avenue
Pasadena, CA 91101

Phone: 310-568-9100

Cloudbreak Communities is the brand name for the family of mission-driven Limited-Liability Companies engaged in the development and operation of service-enriched affordable housing for veterans. Owned and operated by Cantwell-Anderson, Inc., a California Corporation, the various Cloudbreak companies which make up Cloudbreak Communities, have completed the development of nearly 2,899 beds/units in 9 communities across 5 states and partnered numerous public, private and non-profit entities in the operation of supportive services and healthcare within each site. There are currently 3 communities across Arizona, two in Phoenix, one in Prescott.

Victory Place

This 5-acre campus in the South Mountain Village of Phoenix hosts 177 beds comprised of 70 VA Grant and Per Diem transitional housing beds operated by United States Veterans Initiative (U.S. VETS) and 107 units of permanent housing with support services provided by U.S. VETS and the Phoenix VA Healthcare for Homeless Veterans.

Victory Place Phase III

This campus added 75 additional units of permanent housing with support services for homeless and formerly homeless veterans aged 55 and older and features 15 Project-Based Department of Housing and Urban Development Veterans Affairs Supportive Housing (HUD VASH) Vouchers.

These vouchers are used to serve the most vulnerable homeless veterans in the community ensuring no veteran is left behind.

Victory House

Located in the lower wing of the VA Domiciliary, Cloudbreak Phoenix, LLC, negotiated a long-term capital lease with the Northern Arizona VA Healthcare System to purpose unutilized VA space for the transitional housing needs of homeless veterans in rural Arizona. U.S. VETS operates 58 VA Grant and per-diem beds at this location.

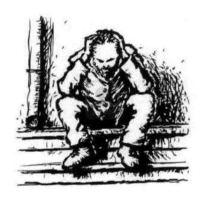

Internet Websites & Resources for Disabled Veterans

*"**From time to time, the tree of liberty must be watered with the blood of tyrants and patriots.**"* - Thomas Jefferson

ADAPTIVE SPORTS WEBSITES

Adaptive Sports Alliance — www.adaptivesportsalliance.com

Disabled Veterans Sports Program — www.sports.yahoo.com/photos/dsabledveterans-sports-program-slideshow

Adaptive Sports Center — www.adaptivesports.org

VA Adaptive Sports Homepage — www.va.gov/adaptivesports program.org

Adaptive Sports Foundation — www.adaptivesportsfoundation.org

Adaptive Sports Equipment — www.adaptivesportsequipment.com

Adaptive Sports — www.disabledsportsusa.org

Paralyzed Veterans Racing — www.pva.org

National Veterans Wheelchair Games — www.wheelchairgames.va.gov

Palaestra — www.palaestra.com

United States Power Soccer Association — www.powersoccerusa.org

National Veterans Wheelchair Games — www.disabledsportsusa.org

Disabled Sports USA Far West — www.dsusafw.org

Disabled Sportsman — www.disabledsportsman.com

Arizona Disabled Sports	www.arizonadisabledsports.com
National Sports Center of the Disabled	www.nscd.org
Disabled World – Disability Sports	www.disabledworld.com/sports
Wounded Warrior Disabled Sports Project Paralympics	www.woundedwarriorproject.org

MOBILITY ISSUE WEBSITES

Mobility Management	www.mobilitymgmt.com
The Mobility Project	www.themobilityproject.com
The Ralph Braun Foundation	www.ralphbraunfoundation.org
The Association for Driver Rehabilitation Specialists	www.driver-ed.org
The Magazine for Active Wheelchair Users	www.newmobility.com
Aquila Corporation-Wheelchair Cushions	www.aquilacorp.com
Portable Vehicle Hand Controls for the Disabled	www.wheelability.com
Veteran Mobility	www.veteranmobility.com
We Care Designs, LLC	www.paraladder.com
Auto Mobility Sales	www.automobilitysales.com
Performance Mobility	www.performancemobility.com
Operation Independence for Veterans	www.vans4vets.com
Ford Mobility Motoring	www.fordmobilitymotoring.comveterans.mob
Proving Practical Solutions for Today's Mobility Challenges	www.veteranhandcontrols.com
Veteran Mobility Information	www.vantagemobilityinc.com
Disabled Sportsman Magazine	www.dsportsman.com
SANDS USA	www.sandsusa.org
Better Life Mobility Center	www.betterlifemobility.com
VMI Mobility Center	www.vmimobilitycenter.com/veterans-program
Brunswick Mobility Professionals	www.brunswickmobility.com/disabled-veterans
Mobility Works	www.mobilityworks.com/veteransassistance.php
Adaptive Mobility Equipment	www.amemobility.com
Veterans Mobility	www.vetmobility.com
Toyota Mobility	www.ToyotaMobility.com

Quantum Power Chairs	www.quantumrehab.com
Freedom Rides Motorcycle Conversions	www.freedomrides.biz
College Park Technology for the Human Race	www.college-park.com
Rush Foot (for Amputees)	www.rushfoot.com
Sleeve Art (for Amputees)	www.fredslegs.com
Ferrier-Coupler, Inc.	www.ferrier.coupler.com
TRS, Inc.	www.trsprosthetics.com
Permobil	www.permobil.com
Abilities365.com	www.abilities365.com
Abilities Expo-The Event for People with Disabilities	www.abilitiesexpo.com
Apex Designs	www.apexq.com
VMI-Wheelchair Cushions	www.vantagemobility.com
New Mobility	www.newmobility.com
AMS Vans, Inc.	www.amsvans.com
Disaboom	www.disaboom.com
Better Life Mobility Center	www.betterlifemobility.com
Mobility Supercenter	www.mobilitysupercenter.com
Ride Away	www.ride-away.com
Adaptive Daily Living Aids	www.wrightstuff.biz
Automotive Mobility Solutions	www.nmeda.com/veterans-disabilities
Agar Enterprises	www.agorenterprises.com
New Mobility	www.newmobility.com
Ability Center – Elevating Your Quality of Life	www.AbilityCenter.com

SPINAL CORD INJURY (SCI)

BACKBONES	www.backbonesonline.com
National SCI Association	www.spinalcord.org
A Program of United Spinal Association	www.usersfirst.org
United Spinal	www.unitedspinal.org
Spinal Cord Injury Support	www.apparalyzed.com
SCI Information	www.spinal-cord.org
SCI and Brain Injury Center	www.brainandspinalcord.org

SCI Support Group	www.scisg.org
Spine Injury Rehabilitation Center	www.stemcellofamerica.com/SI
SCI Recovery	www.scirecovery.com
Christopher & Dana Reeves Foundation	www.christopherreeve.org

TRAVEL FOR THE MILITARY AND THE DISABLED

Travel Discounts for Military and Veteran	www.militaryvacationtravel.com
Disability Travel-Veterans on the Lake	www.veteransonthelake.com
Disabled World-Accessible Disability Travel Information	www.disabled-world.com/travel
Military Cruise Discounts, Military Discounts, Military Travel	www.vacationstogo.com
Able to Travel	www.abletotravel.org
Society of Accessible Travel and Hospitality	www.sath.org
Travel for Disabled	www.travelfordisabled.com
Veteran Travel Resources	www.vettravel.com
Veterans Access Travel Center	www.accesstravelcenter.com /veterans.cfm
Disabled Travelers.Com	www.disabledtravelers.com/veterans.html
Vacation Deals for Veterans and Their Families	www.veteransholidays.com
Military and Veteran Travel Discounts	www.veteransadvantage.com
Disability Travel/Veterans on the Lake	www.veteransonthelakeresort.com
Military and Veteran Discounts	www.localveterandiscounts.com
Discount Travel for Military and Veterans	www.vacationstogo.com/military-discounts.search.cmf
Disabled Veterans National Foundation	www.helpingdisabledvets.com
Dynamic Travel and Cruises	www.dynamictravel.com/veterans
Veterans Travel Service, Inc.	www.vtstvl.com
Resources for Disabled Veterans and Families- Air Travel	www.disabledvetresources.com/resources/air_travel

176

Military Disney Tips	www.militarydisneytips.com/2013-Disney-Armed-Forces-Salute.html
Military Travel Deals	www.americandiscountcruises.com/military-travel
Emerging Horizons – The Accessible Travel Newsletter	www.emerginghorizons.com
Discovery Tours	www.discovery-tours.com
Fun Jet Vacations	www.funjet.com
Get Ski Tickets	www.getskitickets.com
Veteran Vacation Deals	www.veteransholidays.com
Timeshares for Veterans	www.timesharesforveterans.com
Vacations for Veterans	www.vacationsforveterans.org
Bed and Breakfasts for Veterans	www.betterwaytostay.com

DISABLED VETERAN DATING WEBSITES

Dating for the Disabled	www.dating4disabled.com
Operation We Are Here	www.operationwearehere.com
Meet Disabled Singles	www.meetdisabledsingles.com
Disabled Match Making	www.disabledmatchmaking.com
Dating Disabled	www.datingdisabled.com
Disabled Persons	www.disabledpersons.com
Date Disabled	www.datedisabled.com
Disability Dating	www.disabilitydating.com
Whispers 4 U	www.whispers4u.com
Able to Love You	www.abletoloveyou.com
Disabled Singles Dating	www.disabledsinglesdating.com
Dating 4 Disabled	www.dating4disabled.net

CANINE TRAINING

Hero Dogs, Inc.	hero@hero-dogs.org
Paws of Fame	www.patriotpaws.org
Canine Companions for Independence	www.cci.org
Hero Dogs for Wounded Veterans	www.hero-dogs.org
America's Vet Dogs	www.vetdogs.org
Freedom Service Dogs	www.freedomservicedogs.org
Operation We Are Here	www.operationwearehere.com

NEADS-Canines for Combat Veterans www.neads.org
PTSD Service Dogs for Veterans www.operationdeltadog.org
Veterans Service Dog
Program www.theveteransservicedogprogram.com

Canine Angels www.canineangelsservicedogs.org
4 Paws for Veterans www.4pawsforability.org
Shelter Dogs Help Veterans with PTSD www.pawnation
Veterans Moving Forward www.vetsfwd.org
Dogs for Veterans www.dogsforveterans.org
Soldier's Best Friend www.soldiersbestfriend.org
Veteran Service Dogs www.guidedogs.org
Dogs for Vets www.dogsforvets.com
Assistance Dogs for Veterans www.vetshelpingheroes.com
Dogs for Disabled Veterans www.freedomservicedogs.org
(Lake Pleasant website)
Operation Delta Dog www.operationdeltadog.org
Power Paws Assistance Dogs www.azpowerpaws.org
The Guide Horse Foundation www.guidehorse.com
Top Dog www.topdogusa.org
Gabriel's Angels www.gabrielsangels.org
Free My Paws Canine Training www.freemypaws.com
Vets Adopt Pets www.vetsadoptpets.org
Companion Animal Association of Arizona www.caaainc.org
Dogs for Vets www.dogs4vets.org
Vets Helping Heroes www.vetshelpingheros.org
Tower of Hope www.thetowerofhope.org
Land of Pure Gold www.landofpuregold.com
Handi Dogs, Inc. www.handi-dogs.org

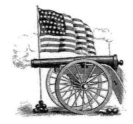

INFORMATION AND RESOURCES

Veterans Disability Website	www.theveterandisability.com
Military Living	www.militaryliving.com
Military and Veteran Benefits	www.military.com
Veteran Owned Business Directory	www.veteransownedbusiness.com
Disabled Veterans Services, Inc.	www.disabledveteransservices.com
Disabled U.S. Veterans	www.disabledusveterans.com
Veterans Financial, Inc.	www.veteransfinancial.com
Dell Computers Veterans Discounts	www.dell.com/veterans
The Disabled Veterans Resource Center	www.disabledveteransresourcecenter.org
Disabled Veteran Resources	www.accessfordisabled.com/disabled_resources
Disabled Veterans National Foundation	www.dvnf.org/resources
Resources for Disabled Veterans and their Families	www.disabledvetresources.com
Veterans Resources	www.veteranresources.org
Free Resources for Disabled American Veterans	www.disabledveteranassistance.org
Disabled Person Resources	www.disabledperson.com/resources
Arizona Military Assistance Mission	www.azmam.org
We Salute	www.wesalute.net
WE Magazine	www.wemagazine.com
Reach Out Magazine	www.reachoutmag.com
Enabled Online	www.enabledonline.com
Emerging Horizons The Accessible Travel Newsletter	www.emerginghorizons.com
Mainstream – Magazine for the Able-Disabled	www.mainstream.mag.com
Disabled Person	www.disabledperson.com
The Ragged Edge Magazine	www.ragged-edge-mag.com
Disability World	www.disabilityworld.com

New Mobility	www.newmobility.com
Disability Resources on the Internet	www.disabilityresources.org
Disability Help Center	www.ssdhelpcenter.org
Arizona Association of Providers for People with Disabilities	www.aappd.org
Discounts for People with Disabilities	www.disableddiscounts.com
Need Help Paying Bills	www.needhelppayingbills.com
ASU Disability Resource Center	www.eoss.asu.edu.drc
Disabled Person	www.disabledperson.com
Amputee Coalition of America	www.amputeecoalition.org
Park Art Ranch	www.nps.gov/pefo
National Park Service	
Grand Canyon National Park	www.nps.gov/grca
Camp Corral for Children of Wounded, Disabled or Fallen Military Soldiers	www.campcorral.org
Vets Helping Service/Service Dogs/Guide Dogs	www.vetshelpingheros.org
The Tower of Hope/Providing Service Dogs for Independent Living	www.thetowerofhope.org
Fun Jet Vacations	www.funjet.com
Get Ski Tickets	www.getskitickets.com
Free Disabled Secrets	www.freedisabledsecrets.com
Veteran Vacation Deals	www.veteransholidays.com
Time Shares for Veterans	www.timesharesforvets.com
Free Internet Resource Links for Veterans	www.gulfwarvets.com/resource.htm
Property Home Grants	www.propertyhomegrants.blogspot.com
Better Life Mobility	www.betterlifemobility.com
Providing Resources to Help Heroes and their Loved Ones	www.familyofavet.com/financial help_forveterans.htm

Helping Hands for Wounded Veterans www.hhwv.org
Veteran Travel Resources www.vettravel.com
Pets for Vets www.pets-for-vets.com
A Tool for Military Members to Securely
Submit their Identity Online to Help Better
Access Discounts and Savings www.id.me

VA Aid and Attendance www.veteransfinancial.com
Kieve Veteran Camp - Free for Operation Iraqi
Freedom & Enduring Freedom Veterans www.kieve.org/veterans

A Site to Help Better Inform Veterans to
Make Better Decisions Concerning their
Benefits www.disabledvet.com

Military and Veteran Discounts www.militaryandveteransdiscounts.com
How to get a Car if you have a
Disability www.wikihow.com/get-a-free-car-
if-you-had-a_disability

Vacations for Veterans www.veteransprograms.com
A Message Forum for Veterans to Help Each
Other Find Assistance & Programs www.veteransprograms.com

Discounts for People with Disabilities www.disableddiscounts.com
Veterans for Advocacy Foundation www.veterans4advocacy.org
United States Veterans Initiative www.usvetsinc.org

Arizona Veterans Service Advisory
Commission http://dvs.az.gov/about/advisory-commission

Disabled Person Resources www.disabledperson.com/resources

Resources for Disabled Veterans www.aahd.us/bestpracticeresources-for
disabled-veterans

Warrior Transition Command/
Disabled Veterans www.wtc.army.mil/soldier/disabled
veterans.html

Disabled Veterans Association
of the U. S. www.asua.org/internetresources/pages/Army/DV.aspx

Your Guide to the Web Since 1995	www.freebyte.com
Arizona Caregivers	www.azcaregivers.org
Uncover the Resources to Achieve	www.educationmoney.com
Enhancing Lives Through Education,	
Support and Experiences	www.archaz.org
Military Discount List	www.militarydiscountlist.com
Arizona Disabled Veteran Foundation	www.advf.org
Amputee Coalition of America	www.amputeecoalition.org
National Park Service	
Grand Canyon National Park	www.nps.gov/grca
Camp Corral for Children	
of Wounded, Disabled or	
Fallen Military Soldiers	www.campcorral.org
Disabled Person Job Board	www.disabledperson.com
Honoring Their Sacrifice, Educating	
Their Legacy	www.foldsofhonor.com
Veterans Advisory Commission	www.scottsdale.az.gov/accessible /resources/physically
Shades of Green at Walt Disney Resort	www.shadesofgreen.org
Cars for Vets	www.vet-cars.com
Pets for Vets	www.pets-for-vets.com
Free Adventure Trips for Veterans	www.182aw.ang.af.mil/news /story.asp?id=123193277
Vetmade Vehicle Donation Program	www.cars4disabledvets.org
Veterans Family United Foundation	www.veteransfamiliesunited.org
RVDreams.com	www.rv-dreams.activeboard.com
Veteran Home Ownership	www.newdayusa.com
Free Disabled Secrets	www.freedisabledsecrets.com
Veteran Artist Network	www.veteranartistnetwork.com
Barrier free Homes for Disabled	
Veterans	www.accessibledreams.org/barrier-free-homes-for-disabled-veterans
Property Home Grants	www.propertyhomegrants.blogspot.com
Helping Hands for Wounded Veterans	www.hhwv.org

Military Order of the Purple Heart, Sierra
Vista Chapter 572   www.moph572.org

Housing and Mortgages   www.mortgageloan.com/veterans for veterans

Military Discounts   www.id.me
Viking Cruise Lines   www.vrc.com
The One-Stop Shop for Your Military
Disability Needs   www.militarydisabilitymade easy.com

American Red Cross for
Southern Arizona   www.redcross.org/southern arizona
PC's for Veterans   www.pcsforvets.com
Cell Phones for Soldiers   www.cellphoneforsoldiers.com
American Military University   www.amuonline.com/veterans
Southwest Veterans Chamber
of Commerce   www.southwestchamber.com
                                   www.southwestveteranschamber.com

Veterans Heritage Project   www.VeteransHeritage.org
U.S. Air Force Information Site   www.BaseOps.net
Military and Veterans
Discounts   www.militaryandveteransdiscounts.com

Segway's for Veterans   www.segways4vets.com
Discounts for Veterans   www.tiphero.com/195-discounts-for-veterans
Veterans Discounts   www.veteransdiscounts.com
Gift Card Granny   www.giftcardgranny.com
Military Discounts   www.thefrugalgirls.com/military-discounts
Legal Assistance   www.LawForVeterans.org
Grants for Disabled Veterans   www.ability-mission.org/grants-disabled
                                         -veterans.html

47 Federal Assistance Grants and Services
for Veterans   www.educationmoney.com

Grants for Veterans   www.grantwatch.com/cat/38/ veterans-grants.html
Grants for Disabled Veterans   www.veteransunited.com
Disabled Veteran Grants   www.grantsforveterans.com

Grants for Veterans (Free Government Money)	www.gofreegovernmentmoney.com/grants_for_veterans
Veteran Grants	www.usgrants.org/veteran- grants.htm
Government Grants and Loans: Disabled Veterans	www.fedmoney.com/grantssu0213.htm
Apply for Home Property Grants- Free and Approved	www.propertyhomegrants.blogspot.com
The Military Wallet	www.themilitarywallet.com/category/deals-discounts
Providing Resources to Help Heroes and their Loved One	www.familyofavet.com/financial_helpveterans.html
Different Types of Grants for Women Veterans	www.governmentgrantspro.com/grants-articles/different-types-of-grants-for-women-veterans-092640.html
That Freebie Site	www.thatfreebiesite.com

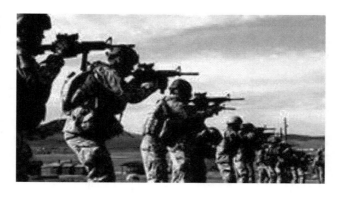

184

Amputee Resources

Today, amputees have access to more information than ever before. The internet plays a significant role by making resources available day or night, regardless of your location. Manufacturer websites, non-profit organizational websites and prosthetic-related message boards offer a wide scope of information about technology, life as an amputee, and healthcare issues. At freedom-innovations.com, they have worked to provide detail about their products and services so that you can make educated choices in collaboration with your prosthetist and healthcare team.

Below is a list of some online resources where you can find more information. You will also find a selection of real-life success stories, detailing the lives and accomplishments of quite an inspiring group of people.

- 360 O&P – is a home for web-based community focused on empowerment and sharing the latest practical information patients and professionals.
- The American Board of Certification in Orthotics, Prosthetics and Pedorthotics – This organization is the national certifying and accrediting body for the orthotic, prosthetic and pedorthotic professions.
- The American orthotic & Prosthetic Association – through government relations efforts, this organization works to raise awareness of the profession and impact policies that affect the future of the O&P industry.
- Adaptive Action Sports – this organization creates programs and opportunities for individuals with permanent physical disabilities to participate in "action sports" and /or the art and music scene that follows them.
- Amputee Coalition of America – this organization reaches out to people with limb loss and empowers them through education, support and advocacy.
- Disabled Sports USA – this organization seeks to provide the opportunity for individuals with disabilities to gain confidence and dignity through participation in sports, recreation and related educational programs.

- Orthotic and Prosthetic Assistance Fund – this organization enables individuals served by the orthotic and prosthetic community to enjoy the rewards of personal achievement, physical fitness and social interaction.

Here is a list of some websites dealing with amputation:

Active Amp	www.activeamp.org
American Academy of Orthotists and Prosthetists	www.oandp.org
American Amputee Foundation, Inc.	www.americanamputee.org
Amputee Coalition	www.amputee-coalition.org
National Amputee Foundation	www.nationalamputation.org
Barr Foundation	www.barrfoundation.org
Limbs for Life Foundation	www.limbsforlife.org
Amputee Resource Foundation of America	www.amputeeresource.org

"Army: A body of Men assembled to rectify the mistakes of the Diplomats" - Josephus Daniels

THE ENTREPRENEURSHIP BOOTCAMP FOR VETERANS WITH DISABILITIES (EBV) PROGRAM

The Institute for Veterans and Families at Syracuse University (IVMF) is the first interdisciplinary national institute in higher education focused on the social. Economic, education and policy issues impacting veterans and their families post-service. Through our focus on veteran-facing programming, research and policy, employment and employer support, and community engagement, the institute provides in-depth analysis of the challenges facing the veteran community, captures best practices and serves as a forum to facilitate new partnerships, and strong relationships between the individuals and organizations committed to making a difference for veterans and military families.

The Entrepreneurship Bootcamp for Veterans with Disabilities National Program is a novel, one-of-a-kind initiative designed to leverage the skills, resources and infrastructure of higher education to offer cutting-edge, experimental training in entrepreneurship and small business management to post 9/11 veterans and their families.

The aim of the program is to open the door to economic opportunity for our veterans and their families by developing their competencies in creating and sustaining an entrepreneurial venture.

EBV National Facts:

- The EBV Consortium represents the first major partnership of America's schools and colleges of business since World War II, formed with the express purpose of serving military veterans.

- Named by Inc. Magazine as one of the '10 Best' entrepreneurship programs in the U.S. (2011).

- EBV was named a 'National Best Practice' for serving veterans and their families by the Secretary of the Army in 2009.

- Awarded the McGraw-Hill Prize from the Academy of Management for the most innovative entrepreneurship program implemented by U.S. business schools in 2010.

For more Information:

EBV National Headquarters
Syracuse University
700 University Avenue
Suite #303
Syracuse, NY 13244
Email: ebvinfo@syr.edu
Phone: 315-443-0141
Fax: 315-443-0312

The Boots to Business Program

You've served your country with great honor. The U.S. Small Business Administration (SBA) is proud to serve you as you start your own business. The Boots to Business Program was developed as part of the U.S. Department of Defense's Transition Assistance Program to educate and train you on the basics of business ownership and to assist you with your entrepreneurial planning. This program is a great first step to being on your way to business ownership or gainful self-employment.

With a network of skilled advisors and partners, they will help you with any questions that you might have, provide follow-up counseling and training, assist you in accessing capital, and advise you on Federal Contracting opportunities. This network includes SBA District Offices, Veteran Business Outreach Centers, Small Business Development Centers, Women's Business Centers, and SCORE* executive mentors. You can find your nearest SBA Office or partner at www.sba.gov/tools/local-assistance.

After a basic introductory two-day course, there is an 8-week, interactive online Foundations of Entrepreneurship Course, which focuses on the fundamentals of developing a business plan. The course is offered at no cost by a consortium of universities led by the Institute for Veterans and Military Families at Syracuse University.

*SCORE is a great place where you can get **FREE** confidential business advice from expert advisors committed to helping you succeed. There are 27 SCORE locations scattered throughout Arizona.

You can go to www.score.org to find out where they are located and if one is near you. On this site, you can also request a mentor or sign-up for one of their many workshops.

CHOOSING A SCHOOL THAT IS RIGHT FOR YOU

As an eligible Service Member, Veteran, Dependent, Guard Member or Reservist planning to use the GI Bill you are a consumer about to make one of the most important decisions of your life. Would you buy a car before considering your needs or before checking available resources for ratings and prices? That is why you owe it to yourself to thoroughly consider your needs before choosing a school or program.

Service Members Opportunity Colleges

Service Members Opportunity Colleges (SOC) was created in 1972 to provide educational opportunities to service members who, because they frequently moved from place to place, had trouble completing college degrees. SOC functions in cooperation with 15 higher education associations, the Department of Defense, and Active and Reserve Components of the Military Services to expand and improve voluntary postsecondary education opportunities for service members worldwide. SOC is funded by the Department of defense through a contract with the American Association of State Colleges and Universities (AASCU).

The contract is managed for DoD by the Defense Activity for Non-Traditional Education Support (DANTES). Visit the SOC website at www.soc.aascu.org.

Here is a list of SOC's in Arizona. The letters in parentheses after each college's name indicate whether it offers associate, bachelor's, master's, and/or doctoral degrees. You can get more information by visiting their websites.

Argosy University, Phoenix **(a, b, m, d)**
Arizona State University **(b, m, d)**
Arizona Western College **(a)**
Art Institute of Phoenix **(a, b)**
Brighton College **(a)**
Chandler-Gilbert Community College **(a)**
Cochise College **(a)**
DeVry University-Glendale Center **(b, m)**
DeVry University-Mesa Center **(a, b, m)**
DeVry University-Phoenix Campus **(a, b, m)**
Dunlap-Stone University **(a, b)**
Estrella Mountain Community College **(a)**
Glendale Community College **(a)**
Grand Canyon **(b, m, d)**
Harrison Middleton University **(a, b, m, d)**
ITT Technical Institute-Phoenix **(a, b)**
ITT Technical Institute-Tempe **(a, b)**
ITT Technical Institute-Tucson **(a, b)**
Mesa Community College **(a)**
Northern Arizona University **(b, m, d)**
Paradise Valley Community College **(a)**
Penn Foster College **(a)**
Phoenix College **(a)**
Pima Community College **(a)**
Prescott College-Adult Degree **(b, m)**
Rio Salado College **(a)**
Scottsdale Community College **(a)**
Sessions College for Professional Design **(a)**
South Mountain Community College **(a)**
University of Arizona South **(b, m, d)**
University of Phoenix **(a, b, m, d)**
Western International University **(a, b, m)**

Veterans Upward Bound Program

One program established to assist veterans with making the transition to higher education is Veterans Upward Bound (VUB), a free U.S. Department of Education (ED) funded program whose primary focus is education. VUB projects help qualifying veterans make the transition from military to civilian life, complete their GED, or enter college or other postsecondary training programs. VUB is an educational and skills program designed specifically to serve the needs of veterans, whether they are from the Vietnam era, the 80's or 90's, or today's combat veterans of Iraq or Afghanistan. The program can be described as 'academic boot camp' and assists veterans in preparing to succeed in the classroom.

For more information about the VUB, and to find the program nearest you, visit their website at www.navub.org.

The following colleges and career schools have a special interest in recruiting veterans.

Embry-Riddle Aeronautical University – is the best choice for military personnel who seek fulfilling and distinguished careers in global security and intelligence, cyber security, aerospace, unmanned aircraft systems, business, aviation, and engineering. If you believe you have what it takes to be number one – to be a leader – don't settle for anything less. Come learn with the best at the top aerospace university in the country.

They offer 18 four-year degrees and two master's degrees, plus minors and concentrations to match your interests. Leading companies and government agencies (Accenture, Boeing, JetBlue, Lockheed Martin, Raytheon, Southwest Airlines, CIA, FBI, National Transportation Safety Board) provide research and internship opportunities around the world.

Admissions Office
3700 Willow Creek Road
Prescott, AZ 8630
928-777-6600
1-800-888-3728 Toll Free
E-mail: pradmit@erau.edu
Website: www.prescott.erau.edu

Military Friendly® Schools

The Military Friendly® assessment process includes extensive research and required completion of a proprietary, data-driven survey.
All Military Friendly® surveys, methodology, criteria and weightings were developed with the assistance of an independent Advisory Board composed of higher education and recruitment professionals from across the country.

Here is a list of Military Friendly® Schools throughout the State of Arizona.

Arizona State University - **www.asu.edu**
Arizona State University – Skysong/Online - **www.skysong.asu.edu**
Arizona Summit Law School - **www.azsummitlaw.edu**
Arizona Western College - **www.azwestern.edu**
Central Arizona College - **www.centralaz.edu**
Chandler-Gilbert Community College - **www.cgc.maricopa.edu**
Cochise College - **www.cochise.edu**
Embry-Riddle Aeronautical University – Prescott – **www.prescott.erau.edu**
Estrella Mountain Community College - **www.estrellamountain.edu**
Grand Canyon University - **www.gcu.edu**
HDS Truck Driving Institute - **www.hdatruckdrivinginstitute.com**
Mesa Community College - **www.mesacc.edu**
Motorcycle Mechanics Institute - **www.uti.edu**
New Horizons Southern California and Southern Arizona - **www.nhsocal.com or www.nhsoaz.com**
Northern Arizona University (NAU) - **www.nau.edu**
Ottawa University - **www.ottawa.edu/locations/adult-and-online locations/phoenix-location**
Southwest Truck Driver Training, Inc.- **www.swtdt.com**
The Art Institute of Phoenix - **www.artinstitutes.edu/phoenix**
The Refrigeration School, Inc. - **www.refrigerationschool.com**
The University of Arizona – Main Campus - **www.ua.edu**
The W. A. Franke College of Business – Northern Arizona University - **www.franke.nau.edu**
TTY Career College - **www.ttycareercollege.edu**
Universal Technical Institute - **www.uti.edu**
University of Advancing Technology - **www.uat.edu**

You can visit their websites to learn more about what they have to offer our military. Programs like Military Scholarships, Military Tuition Discounts, In-State Tuition for Military Spouses & Dependents, Credit for Military Training and many more worthwhile military programs.

"It was the soldier, not the reporter, who has given us freedom of the press.

It is the soldier, not the poet, who has given us freedom of speech.

It is the soldier, not the campus organizer, who has given us the freedom to demonstrate.

It is the soldier, who salutes the flag, who serves beneath the flag, and whose coffin is draped by the flag, who allows the protester to burn the flag."

- Unknown

Grants

"Discipline is the soul of an army. It makes small numbers formidable; procures success to the weak, and esteem to all."
– Gen. George Washington

There could be no denying the fact that getting government grants for people with disabilities is actually quite simple. Of course, it is like building a wall. In general, laying a brick is quite simple but laying so many bricks is not no easy. More to the point, just getting the accurate information is enough to get you started. For your knowledge, there are two major types of disabled grants, one for personal use and the other one for the business purpose. Just spending some time over the web will give you relevant information on how to get these grants online.

If this is the first time you are going to apply for a grant, then you will need to take the assistance of a professional who can help you out. First and foremost, you need to find a granting agency that you feel comfortable working with. You are also recommended to conduct a comprehensive research before you choose one you think that suits you the best. Grants for disabled war veterans are also provided by the federal government, thus if you or a friend of yours has been injured during war, you should surely apply for a grant since there is no one as deserving as you.

The great news is that the disability grants are part of the millions of dollars the federal government keeps aside for the funds and people with any kind of disability usually make the cut.

If you are among the ones who are physically challenged, then you can surely get a grant. As a matter of fact, there are millions of dollars that are provided each year as free grants and there is no reason why you should not be one of the privileged few. One of the best things about this funding assistance for the disabled people, like all other grants, is that they do not have to be repaid. Aside from getting a significant amount of cash, you can also get an opportunity to use the government grants that are related to counseling, equipment, books, etc.

195

In the market, you can spot a grant for just about any disability and they all will assist you to make your world a much more accessible and enjoyable place.

Are you in need of some extra money? Have you lost your job recently or taking a very little amount to your home, in the way of a salary? If this is the case, help is at hand, direct from government sponsored institutions. No matter the financial burden you are experiencing, the government comes forward to distribute millions of dollars every year for low income households, with types of grants ranging from minority government grants to scholarships for higher education as well.

A huge number of folk's search for the ways of getting these government grants, but only a few are aware of how to apply for them.

All in all, it is not even uncommon to find disabled grants available for fulfilling varied purposes of the people with disabilities, and there are ways of ensuring your grant application always gets approved.

The United States government and Arizona's Office of Finance has set aside $14,479,000 in federal grants and $12,997,000 in other types of government financial assistance for people who reside in the state of Arizona. As long as you have a valid citizenship card (a green card) or a permanent resident certificate, you may be eligible to apply and receive Arizona government grants.

Government financial aid in Arizona is distributed to various economic sectors, with the majority of the budget in business, education (Pell and college grants), housing, veteran, and personal grants.

Arizona Veteran Grants – Residents of Arizona who have entered or who are currently active duty military, naval, and air force are eligible to claim and receive government funding in the form of veteran grants. Arizona resident veterans may be eligible to apply for various types of veteran grants and benefits. According to the local military office in Arizona, to eligible for veteran grants:

- you must be a veteran who enlisted in the military, naval force, or air force, before September 7, 1980, *__OR__*
- you must be a veteran who enlisted in the military, naval force, or air force, after September 7, 1980, with at least 24 months of active duty time.

Veterans Health Care Benefits – All veterans in

Arizona are eligible to apply for additional health care benefits provided by the federal government. There are currently 532,206 veterans in the state of Arizona – 477,985 male veterans and 54,221 female veterans. They will be able to receive veteran health care grants as long as they are eligible for veteran health care benefits.

The United States government offers health benefits to active and discharged veterans and their dependents. The VA honors veterans of all eras for their courage and sacrifice by providing comprehensive medical benefits package to promote, preserve, or restore good health.

Veteran Grants for Disabled Veterans – For

veterans who have suffered permanent injuries during historical or active wars are eligible to apply and receive Veteran Grants for Disabled Veterans offered by the military office in Arizona.

There are currently more than 425,067 veterans in Arizona who are "war-time" veterans, which means they have been involved in one of the following wars:

- more than 159,896 of the 425,067 soldiers entered and survived in the Gulf War
- more than 185,867 of the 425,067 soldiers entered and survived the Vietnam War
- more than 53,727 of the 425,067 soldiers entered and survived the Korean Conflict
- more than 25,577 of the 425,067 soldiers entered and survived World War II.

And just as important, there are currently 130,255 "peace-time" veterans as well.

The Office of Finance and Economic Growth in Arizona has set aside governmental funding for grants in education, small business, and housing only to qualified veterans in the state of Arizona. It does not matter if you are a "war-time" veteran or a "peace-time" veteran, there are veteran grants available for everyone who has participated or is currently enlisting in the military, naval force, and/or air force.

For example, veterans in Arizona are not only eligible to apply for small business grants that are available to all residents of Arizona, they are also eligible to apply for small business grants for veterans as well. And the same is true for housing and education grants.

Veteran Small Business Grants for Entrepreneurs

– The Department of Veterans Affairs (VA) has created a dedicated Center for Veterans Enterprise (CVE). The purpose of the program is to assist veterans in starting and expanding their business ventures by fostering entrepreneurs with financial support to promote veteran-owned businesses. In addition to small business grants offered by the Small Business Administration (SBA), veterans are also eligible to apply and receive business grants from CVE.

The Arizona Office of Finance and Economic Growth has set aside governmental funding in education grants, small business grants, and housing grants only to qualified veterans in the state of Arizona. It does not matter if you are a "war-time" veteran or a "peace-time" veteran, there are grants available for everyone who has served or is currently serving in the military, naval force, and/or air force.

For example, veterans in Arizona are not only eligible to apply for small business grants that are available to all Arizona residents, but they are also eligible to apply for small business grants for veterans as well and the same holds true for housing grants and education grants.

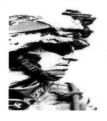

Government Grants for Homeless Veterans – Veteran housing grants are awarded to veterans for construction, acquisition, and renovation of real estate properties. The veteran housing grant initiative also provides financial aid for transportation by helping veterans to purchase vehicles. According to the Housing and Economic Recovery Act, the amount in veteran housing grants will remain unchanged this fiscal year. Specially Adapted Housing (SAH) grants are also available to veterans or service members who have service-connected disabilities to ensure a barrier-free living environment for disabled veterans and service members.

Veteran Education Grants – Veterans and their dependents are eligible to apply and receive veteran education grants. The United States government has launched the Survivor's and Dependents' Educational Assistance Program (DEA) which will provide financial assistance for higher education not only to the veteran but also to applicable dependents as well.

Please note that the funding for dependents will usually last until the date of death of the beneficial veteran.

- Veteran education grants are offered for (not limited to) the following coverage:
- Partial tuition discount or full coverage to undergraduate and graduate program
- 100% participant in the VA's Yellow Ribbon Program
- Credit for CLEP and DSSST examinations
- Financial aid for military training, studies, and experience

The United States government has set aside $14,479,000 in government grants and $12,997,000 in other form of governmental financial funding across all the states to eligible applicants. Veterans who currently residing in the state of Arizona may be eligible to apply for various types of veteran grants and benefits. According to the local military office in Arizona, to eligible for veteran grants:

- You must be a veteran who was enlisted in military, naval force, or air force, before September 7, 1980, **or**
- You must be veteran who enlisted in the military, naval force, or air force, after September 7, 1980 with at least 24 months of active duty.

Arizona Commission for Postsecondary Education
2020 North Central Ave
Suite #650
Phoenix, AZ 85004

Arizona Department of Education
1535 W. Jefferson Street
Phoenix, AZ 85007
602-542-4361
1-800-352-4558 Toll Free

Dr. April L. Osborn
Executive Director

Tom Horne
Superintendent of Public Instruction

Judi Sloan
Communications Specialist

Margaret Dugan
Deputy Superintendent of Public Instruction
Email: ADEINBOX@azed.gov

Contacts:

Email: jsloan@azhighered.gov
Email: cwilliams@highered.gov
Website: http://azhighered.gov

Arizona Educational Grants – Education plays an important role in Arizona. The federal administration in Arizona invests over $10,538,885,516 dollars per year in elementary and secondary institutions alone. Education grants are available for students or even teachers in Arizona to complete and enhance their level of education. Students enrolled in Arizona schools can look into education grants in addition to scholarships. Educational costs can be very, very expensive. Although there are student loans available, students should look into education grants first. Unlike loans, students do not have to pay back the amount they receive in grants.

Teachers in Arizona need to constantly stay on top of new material. Most teachers need to study part-time while teaching full-time at their regular day jobs in schools.

200

Whether you are a college or graduate student, or a teacher or professor who is looking to pursue higher education, you can apply for Arizona Education Grants by submitting a Free Application for Federal Student Aid (FAFSA). The Office of FAFSA in Arizona ensures all eligible residents in Arizona can benefit from federally funded financial aid for education.

The Arizona State Grant Agency provides information on grants, scholarships, and other financial aid for college students, including federally supported state programs such as Byrd scholarships and LEAP (Leveraging Educational Assistance Partnership) grants.

Arizona Small Business Grants – Starting and running and managing a small business in Arizona can be a risky thing to do. To help be successful, you have to do some research. You will need to look into as many funding sources as possible. With more than $14,479,000 in grants and additional local government funding sources of $12,997,000, the majority of the federal budget in government grants is put into the business sector every year as small businesses and large corporations are the foundation of the economic growth in Arizona.

Although the federal government does not publicly provide grants for starting nag expanding a small business, in Arizona, some small business grants are given to business owners to start and grow their ventures, and grant recipients do not have to pay back the funding from the government. Therefore, it makes sense to look into small business grants as one of your sources of funding your business.

Arizona Housing Grants – At an average value of $215,000 per housing property, there are around 2,840,000 real estate properties in Arizona. With an average annual household income of $50,958, less than 69.10% of the people actually paid off their mortgages. A good portion of the residents in Arizona cannot afford to pay off their mortgages.

The Department of Finance has set aside financial aid in the form of housing grants to the people in need, especially if you work at home.

The Office of Departmental Grants Management and Oversight (ODGMO) is responsible for housing grants (HUD Programs and Initiatives) in the state of Arizona. Although there are funds available to Arizona residents, not everyone is eligible to apply and receive Arizona Housing Grants. The ODGMO has a list of policy priorities.

Housing Grants for Low-Income Residents –

Arizona's local government has set aside financial assistance for residents with no or low-income. The main imitative behind this policy is to assist those residents financially while they look for jobs or improve their income.

Housing Grants for Green Homes – The local

government in Arizona actively promotes green indicatives in the housing sector. Funds are available for residents to improve the sustainability of their homes through energy-efficient, environmentally friendly, and healthy design. For metropolitan and some regional areas, housing grants are also given to households to improve location efficiency and disaster resiliency.

Housing Grants for Minorities – To overcome

discrimination due to race, color, nationality, gender, religion, disability, or familial status, the Department of Housing in Arizona actively promotes fair housing by providing financial assistance in the form of housing grants. If you use your home as a platform for improving other outcomes, such as business, education, health, or environment, the HUD Indicatives will be able to provide you with the funding you need.

Arizona Personal Grants – The local state

government in Arizona does not offer financial aid to its residents for personal needs such as getting out of debt, financing a vehicle, etc. But, Arizona residents are eligible to apply for personal grants to receive financial aid to carry out a public purpose of support or stimulation to the economy.

Most people are confused about personal grants. If you are looking for personal financial assistance such as supplemental security income, Medicaid, or state social services, you should look into government benefits instead. Personal grants are financial aid from the local government for its residents under certain circumstances – the use of the financial funding must have a meaningful purpose to the local economy and the economy of Arizona.

Personal Grants for Work at Home Residents
With the aid from the federal government, the Department of Finance and Economic Growth is able to provide financial support to residents who work at home.

To be eligible, you must be a resident of Arizona and have a registered business in Arizona. If your business is in one of the following areas:

- medicine
- education
- scientific research
- technology development

You have a higher chance of getting your grant application approved!

Personal Grants for Education for Residents of Arizona
– Not all students or teachers are eligible to apply for personal education grants. As you do not have to pay back the amount of the grant given to you; Arizona's Office of Education ensures that personal grants are only given to individuals who need financial assistance for their education related to medicine, education, scientific research, and/or technology development. And recipients must use their new knowledge and skill set to improve the local economy and the economy of Arizona.

Personal Grants for Veterans
– If you have served in or are currently on active duty in the military, naval force, or air force, you are eligible to apply for veteran personal grants as long as the funds are being used to stimulate the economy.

You can look at personal grants as "government grants for individuals." Therefore, there are many types of personal grants such as personal housing grants. If an individual has received a grant from the government, he or she has received a type of "personal grant".

Arizona Commission for Postsecondary Education
2020 North Central Ave
Suite #650
Phoenix, AZ 85004

Arizona Department of Education
1535 W. Jefferson Street
Phoenix, AZ 85007
602-542-4361
1-800-352-4558 Toll Free

Dr. April L. Osborn
Executive Director

Tom Horne
Superintendent of Public Instruction

Judi Sloan
Communications Specialist

Margaret Dugan
Deputy Superintendent of Public Instruction
Email: ADEINBOX@azed.gov

Contacts:

Email: jsloan@azhighered.gov
Email: cwilliams@highered.gov
Website: http://azhighered.gov

About the Author

Derek Simmons joined the U.S. Army in 1980. During his 14-year military career, he was able to travel the world. Being assigned to several overseas bases like Giessen and Friedberg, both in Germany and doing a stint in Seoul, South Korea. He served in Saudi Arabia during Operation Restore Freedom and in Somalia during Operations Restore Hope and Continue Hope. With several stateside assignments under his belt, he was finally stationed at Fort Huachuca, Arizona, when a horrific accident ended his military career.

Even with great effort and determination, he was unable to convince the U.S. Army and the U.S. Department of Defense that he was ready to re-enter active duty. Derek was medically retired from the military in 1999. Unable to work due to his disabilities, Derek has been giving it his full attention to learning all he can about what benefits and entitlements are out there for active duty military personnel, veterans and veterans with disabilities in the state of Arizona and has compiled it here in his first book.

Derek is a proud father of a great son and two beautiful and wonderful daughters. And now he is a grandfather of five great little boys. Derek currently resides in Sierra Vista, Arizona, being there now for twenty-three years.

Made in the USA
Lexington, KY
10 November 2019